W9-BEK-896

The Medicine Show

Completely Revised and Updated

The Medicine Show

Consumers Union's practical
guide to some everyday health
problems and health products

By the Editors of Consumer Reports Books

Pantheon Books, New York

The Medicine Show is a Consumer Reports Book published by Consumers Union, the nonprofit organization that publishes CONSUMER REPORTS, the monthly magazine of test reports, product Ratings, and buying guidance. Established in 1936, Consumers Union is chartered under the Not-For-Profit Corporation Law of the State of New York.

The purposes of Consumers Union, as stated in its charter, are to provide consumers with information and counsel on consumer goods and services, to give information and assistance on all matters relating to the expenditure of the family income, and to initiate and to cooperate with individual and group efforts seeking to create and maintain decent living standards.

Consumers Union derives its income solely from the sale of CONSUMER REPORTS and other publications. Consumers Union accepts no advertising and is not beholden in any way to any commercial interest. Its Ratings and reports are solely for the information and use of the readers of its publications.

Neither the Ratings nor the reports nor any other Consumers Union publications, including this book, may be used in advertising or for any commercial purpose of any nature. Consumers Union will take all steps open to it to prevent or to prosecute any such uses of its material or of its name or the name of CONSUMER REPORTS.

Copyright © 1955, 1956, 1957, 1958, 1959, 1960, 1961, 1962, 1963, 1967, 1968, 1970, 1971, 1973, 1974, 1975, 1976, 1977, 1978, 1979, 1980 by Consumers Union of United States, Inc., Mount Vernon, New York 10550

All rights reserved under International and Pan-American Copyright Conventions. Published in the United States by Pantheon Books, a division of Random House, Inc., New York, and simultaneously in Canada by Random House of Canada Limited, Toronto.

Originally published by Consumers Union of United States, Inc., 1961; Second edition 1963; Third edition 1971; Fourth edition 1974, updated September 1976; Fifth edition 1980. This edition of *The Medicine Show* has been published by Pantheon Books for distribution in the book trade.

Library of Congress Cataloging in Publication Data
Main entry under title:

The Medicine show.

Includes index.
1. Medicine, Popular. 2. Quacks and quackery.
3. Health products. I. Consumers Union of United
States. II. Consumer reports.
RC81.M496 1980   615'.856   78–20413
ISBN 0–394–51106–9
ISBN 0–394–73887–X pbk.

Manufactured in the United States of America   8765432

Preface

This fifth edition of *The Medicine Show,* like the earlier ones, is based on articles originally published in the pages of *Consumer Reports,* the monthly magazine of Consumers Union. Such material has been extensively reworked, updated, and expanded. Some chapters contained in previous editions have been dropped, and new chapters have been included. Over the years, Consumers Union has had the expert advice and technical assistance of many consultants who helped develop and revise this material.

Chief among the consultants and principally responsible for the contents of the first and second editions of *The Medicine Show* (1961, 1963) was Consumers Union's medical adviser, Harold Aaron, M.D. In 1967, Marvin M. Lipman, M.D., became medical adviser of Consumers Union and together with Aaron assisted with the third and fourth revisions (1971, 1974). For this edition, Lipman has served as chief consultant.

Lipman is a diplomate of the American Board of Internal Medicine, certified in endocrinology and metabolism, a fellow of the American College of Physicians, a member of the Endocrine Society and of the American Federation for Clinical Research, and clinical associate professor of medicine at New

York Medical College. He serves as consumer liaison to the Miscellaneous External Medication Panel of the Food and Drug Administration's (FDA) Over-the-Counter (OTC) Drug Review Program.

Aaron has been medical adviser of Consumers Union since its founding in 1936. He is a diplomate of the American Board of Internal Medicine, and a fellow of the New York Academy of Medicine, of the New York Academy of Sciences, and of the American Public Health Association. He is also chairman of the editorial board of *The Medical Letter* (see below). The editor of *The Medical Letter*, Mark Abramowicz, M.D., has been a consultant on this edition of *The Medicine Show*.

A number of publications were consulted in the preparation of *The Medicine Show*. Basic sources, frequently cited in this edition, include *The Pharmacological Basis of Therapeutics*, a pharmacology, toxicology, and therapeutics text for physicians and medical students, edited by Louis S. Goodman, M.D., and Alfred Gilman, Ph.D., 5th edition (Macmillan); *AMA Drug Evaluations*, 3rd edition (Department of Drugs, American Medical Association); *Handbook of Nonprescription Drugs*, 6th edition (American Pharmaceutical Association); and *The Medical Letter*, a nonprofit periodical for medical professionals containing evaluations of medical drugs in terms of effectiveness, safety, and possible alternatives.

Also used as references have been the published reports of the FDA's OTC Drug Review Program. Inaugurated in 1972, this extensive study is being conducted by advisory panels of medical and scientific authorities (with an industry and a consumer representative assigned to each panel). The panels have been charged by the FDA with the responsibility of reviewing and evaluating all active ingredients used in approximately 300,000 nonprescription drug products. These ingredients were divided into seventeen therapeutic categories (such as cough and cold medications, pain relievers, skin remedies, etc.) with an advisory panel assigned to each category. Also included for review by the panels were the labeling claims and other statements relevant to these drugs, such as warnings and directions for use. The panel recommendations, which are not binding on the FDA, are published in the *Federal Register* in order to solicit consumer and industry comment. After public comments have been evaluated, the FDA then publishes a tentative final monograph in the *Federal Register* in order to once again invite public reaction. Evaluation of the second series of public comments leads eventually to the final monograph, which has the effect of law. From panel recommendations to monograph, the process may take from two to five years. As of November 1979, twelve panels had published their recommendations and four monographs had been published in final form.

The Medicine Show includes frequent references to products by brand name, usually in discussions of specific products. In general discussions, brand names—particularly of drugs, both prescription and OTC—are mentioned as examples and for ease of identification. For example, a widely prescribed anticoagulant is referred to in the text as "warfarin (Athrombin-K, Coumadin, Panwarfin)"; warfarin is the drug's generic name and in parentheses are the names of some brands of warfarin. Such references are not intended as a comprehensive listing of all brands available. For identification purposes the brand names of prescription drugs are capitalized while brand names of OTC drugs are capitalized and italicized.

As with the fourth edition of *The Medicine Show,* this edition also includes a glossary of select words and phrases related to health and medicine. We urge readers to use the glossary for a better understanding not only of this book but of medical language that may be encountered elsewhere.

Contents

Introduction

Many "everyday health problems" are more annoying than dangerous, more a bother than a threat. Left to their own devices, most people would be quite capable of coping with such problems. But people are not let alone. Indeed, they are all but overwhelmed by "news" stories of miraculous medical discoveries, testimonials—some gratuitous, some paid—from satisfied users, broadcast commercials, print advertisements, and label claims on thousands of products filling the shelves of drugstores and supermarkets. Not only is their peace disturbed; often their money is wasted. And sometimes their very health is threatened.

It is truly a medicine show. No one questions the energy, the ingenuity, or the skill of its promoters. Nor are they all crude hawkers of snake oil; some of the sales pitches are positively low-keyed. What thoughtful consumers should challenge is the extent to which the hucksters succeed in becoming the medical educators of the buyers. The education takes a predictable form. Virtually all promoters of health products proceed in the same pattern: Since selling is their prime purpose, they state no more than what is in their interest. All too often it is in their interest to exploit concern about some aspect of health, real or imagined—for which their bottle, jar, or tube contains the promised answer.

Huckstering should not be confused with education, particularly education on matters of health and medicine. Yet for many people that seems to be the case. In 1972 the Food and Drug Administration reported the results of a study of American health practices and opinions. Those surveyed were presented with the statement that advertisements about medications and health aids "must be true or they wouldn't be allowed to say them." Thirty-eight percent of those surveyed—representing 50 million Americans eighteen and over—agreed with the statement.

Reliable information on health and medicine is needed, and Consumers Union looks to the time when responsible drug advertising will better meet that need. Meanwhile, this book offers consumers "a restorative of balance and perspective, an antidote to excesses, and a purgative for much nonsense" (as stated in 1961 in the first edition of *The Medicine Show*).

Completely revised and brought up to date, this latest edition is intended to help consumers better understand the differences between genuine advances in health and medicine and the sometimes distorted claims of the sellers.

The ailments do not change much from year to year, and neither do the remedies. Old familiar "miracles" of drug advertising still burst upon the scene, only to fade away and be replaced by new ones. Regulations catch up with deceptions. New fads replace old ones. Fresh claims are cranked out to beguile the consumer.

But not all consumers are "believers"; many still refuse to accept the hucksters' medicine show at face value. Like Consumers Union, they question the propriety and the quality of drug advertising as a source of information about health and medicine. This new edition of *The Medicine Show*, like the earlier ones, is addressed not only to these skeptics and truth-seekers, but also to those who may still be susceptible to the blandishments of the hucksters.

The Medicine Show seeks to help consumers make better choices—when choices are available—in many areas of health and medicine. In addition to the familiar world of over-the-counter drugs, the book offers some insights into the puzzling world of prescription drugs, where the pharmaceutical company provides, the physician prescribes, the pharmacist fulfills, and the patient—the consumer—pays and has little or no say.

The thinking of many consultants to Consumers Union—physicians and other health professionals—is represented here, and health professionals should find the book a useful adjunct to their efforts to give their patients sound guidance in medical matters. But *The Medicine Show* is not primarily for health professionals, nor even for patients. It is above all for consumers who want a source of health information significantly more reliable than the next television commercial.

1
Aspirin
and its competitors

Aspirin, in all its various disguises, is the most common of all over-the-counter (OTC) medications. It can be bought plain or buffered, in effervescent tablets or powders, alone or in combination with other analgesics, antacids, antihistamines, and decongestants, and in countless "special" remedies highly touted for arthritis and rheumatism. One day aspirin may be available in liquid form, too. Sales of analgesic products already run more than $700 million a year—an amount exceeded only by that spent for OTC cold and cough items.

Although the number and quantity of inert ingredients used in the formulation and manufacture of aspirin tablets may vary among pharmaceutical companies, Consumers Union believes that there are no well-substantiated differences in clinical effectiveness among standard 5-grain, 325 milligram (mg) brands of aspirin tablets, plain or buffered. The only practical difference is price. *Any* brand of this widely used drug can be an effective remedy for symptomatic relief as an antipyretic and an analgesic in a variety of common ailments. It reduces fever and aches in common respiratory infections such as colds, grippe, and flu, and relieves tension headaches and joint and muscle aches, as well as mild menstrual cramps. For some people it even works as a mild sedative. And, for many patients with chronic rheumatoid arthritis, it is just about as effective in reducing inflammation and swelling of joints as cortisone or its steroid analogues—and is far safer. Aspirin is also a mainstay in the treatment of the more common osteoarthritis.

On the debit side, too, all aspirin is pretty much the same. Really severe pain, such as that experienced by migraine sufferers, is usually not relieved by this drug, either alone or in combination with other OTC analgesic agents. A few people are truly allergic to aspirin and may react with hives or asthma. Such allergic persons should, of course, avoid aspirin in any form or combination (see page 27). Some people may find that aspirin upsets the stomach, particularly when used frequently or in large doses.

Chronic use of aspirin or products containing aspirin, most likely because of the irritative effect on the stomach lining, occasionally may provoke a severe hemorrhage. More commonly, such usage may lead to iron-deficiency anemia. This anemia is due to daily loss, over a long period of time, of small amounts of blood—too small to be discernible—in the stool. There is some evidence that the use of buffered aspirin minimizes this side effect. Enteric-coated aspirin (such as *A.S.A. Enseals* and *Ecotrin*) has a specially formulated outer coating that retards disintegration in the stomach, thereby lessening the chance of such irritation. The product is not foolproof, however; on occasion, whole tablets may be found in the stool. Long-term users of aspirin products require periodic blood counts (every few months) so that their physicians can determine the need for possible iron replacement.

One form of aspirin—chewing gum—is not recommended by Consumers Union's medical consultants. *Aspergum* has been advertised "for minor sore throat pain"; yet aspirin is devoid of any topical anesthetic action. Any benefit derived from this type of preparation can come only from its absorption into the bloodstream from the intestinal tract once the saliva/ aspirin mixture is swallowed. One piece of *Aspergum* contains about two-thirds of the aspirin content in the usual 5-grain tablet. It would be more effective (and cheaper) to swallow a 5-grain aspirin tablet—and then, if you must, to chew a piece of "sugarless" gum. A Food and Drug Administration (FDA) advisory panel on internal analgesics has warned against the use of chewable aspirin and aspirin-containing gum during the week following any oral surgery, including tonsillectomy. CU's medical consultants advise against the use of gargles containing aspirin and say it is far more effective for relief of sore throat discomfort to stick to the traditional remedy: Gargling with warm salt water (see Chapter 3). Not only is aspirin ineffective for the relief of a painful throat, but particles of the tablet may actually cause injury if they are not swallowed and remain in contact with the inflamed membranes of a sore throat.

Pharmacies and other retail stores often sell unadvertised or "house" brands of aspirin at prices ranging from 29 cents to 69 cents per hundred. Until well-controlled studies suggest otherwise, CU knows of no reason to buy anything but the least expensive brand. To command a higher price, manufacturers rely on several million dollars' worth of advertising and some add one or more ingredients to convince the public that they offer something better than plain old aspirin.

In fact, in March 1973 the Federal Trade Commission (FTC) issued orders to three manufacturers of ten leading analgesic products and to their five advertising agencies to halt what the FTC alleged were misleading advertising claims. However, Glenbrook (the makers of *Bayer Aspirin, Bayer Children's Aspirin, Cope, Midol,* and *Vanquish*), Bristol-Myers (the makers of *Bufferin, Excedrin,* and *Excedrin P.M.*), and Whitehall (the makers of *Anacin* and *Arthritis Pain Formula*) denied the allegations and called unconstitutional the FTC proposal that the manufacturers be compelled to correct any misrepresentations.

After examining the documents submitted by the makers of *Bufferin,* the FTC found no reasonable basis for the claim that *Bufferin* works "twice as fast as aspirin." Buffered aspirin, which includes small amounts of antacid, has been shown to be somewhat more rapidly absorbed into the bloodstream than unbuffered aspirin. *Bufferin's* maker exploited these tests as substantiation for its claim. But in 1971 the Panel on Drugs for Relief of Pain of the National Academy of Sciences–National Research Council (NAS–NRC) called that claim "ambiguous and misleading." While recognizing the possibility of slightly faster absorption, the panel concluded that "there is no evidence to indicate that the speed of onset of analgesic action is significantly increased." Furthermore, a study has shown that generic buffered aspirin—much less expensive than *Bufferin*—dissolves as fast as the name brand.

Bufferin has claimed that it "helps prevent the stomach upset often caused by aspirin," ostensibly because it includes, besides the usual amount of aspirin, very small amounts of two common antacids. The NAS–NRC panel reported that most studies it evaluated showed "little difference in the incidence or intensity of subjective gastrointestinal side effects after ingestion of *Bufferin* or plain aspirin."

The panel, in short, found no convincing support for claims that *Bufferin* is either "faster" or "gentler" than straight aspirin. (*Arthritis Strength Bufferin* is like *Bufferin,* except that it contains 50 percent more aspirin per tablet and slightly more of the antacids—see table on pages 22–23.) The FDA advisory panel on internal analgesics concluded in 1977 that buffered aspirin labeling, like that of plain aspirin, should warn against its use by people with stomach problems.

Those in pain are often persuaded by the ads to buy "shotgun" remedies containing many ingredients—apparently on the theory that if there are enough ingredients, at least one might work. At one time, the combination of aspirin, phenacetin, and caffeine, known as the *A.P.C.* tablet, enjoyed considerable popularity, but it is no longer widely sold. By formulating a similar shotgun preparation containing aspirin, acetanilid, and caffeine, *Anacin* entered its bid for the aspirin jackpot. The ads announced that *Anacin* was "like a doctor's prescription," containing not just one or two but three ingredients. When acetanilid was shown to cause certain blood disturbances, *Anacin* substituted phenacetin. Later, when kidney problems were linked with use of phenacetin, it too was dropped from the *Anacin* formulation.

Citing the growing evidence for a relationship between kidney damage and phenacetin in combination drugs, Canada in June 1973 banned the sale of drugs that combined phenacetin with salicylates. Denmark, England, and Sweden have limited the availability on the OTC market of analgesic preparations containing phenacetin. Since 1964 the FDA has taken note of the hazards of phenacetin by requiring a warning on labels of all preparations containing the drug. In the opinion of the FDA advisory panel on internal analgesics, the evidence relating phenacetin to severe kidney problems is derived from a world body of published reports so numerous that the possibility of coincidence is negligible. The FDA has now required that phenacetin be removed from the OTC drug market. CU's medical consultants urge consumers not to buy analgesic combinations that include phenacetin in their formulation (and to dispose of any in the home medicine cabinet).

With phenacetin dropped from the formulation, *Anacin* currently contains only aspirin and caffeine. The amount of caffeine in an *Anacin* tablet is about as much as that in a quarter-cup of brewed coffee. There is no evidence, declares *AMA Drug Evaluations,* that a small dose of caffeine "has an analgesic effect or that it affects the activity of the analgesic components." Thus the only effective analgesic in *Anacin* is aspirin, the anonymous "pain-reliever doctors recommend most for headaches," as the old *Anacin* ads put it.

Anacin is the most heavily promoted single product in the entire OTC market. In September 1978, the FTC called "false" *Anacin* ads claiming that the product was more effective than other analgesics sold OTC for relieving pain. Such a claim, according to the FTC, was not only false but also unfair to consumers, "since the greater effectiveness of *Anacin* has not been scientifically established." Also held to be false was the claim that a person could expect relief from headache pain within twenty-two seconds after taking *Anacin*. "*Anacin*'s analgesic ingredient," the FTC declared, "is not unusual, special or stronger than aspirin, since it is nothing more than aspirin . . . the only other ingredient being caffeine." The FDA panel questioned the inclusion of caffeine: "Its contribution to pain relief has not been shown."

An *Anacin* tablet contains 6.17 grains (400 mg) of aspirin instead of the usual 5 grains (325 mg). A tablet of *Anacin* sells at almost four times the price of a 5-grain tablet of ordinary low-cost aspirin. This is a high premium to pay for an additional 1.17 grains (75 mg) of aspirin per tablet plus the amount of caffeine in a quarter-cup of coffee. (The makers of *Anacin* also market *Arthritis Pain Formula* analgesic tablets; each tablet contains 7.5 grams—486 mg—of aspirin.)

If three ingredients are good, four must be better—at least from an advertising standpoint. So enter *Excedrin*—whose formulation until recently included four ingredients.

One of *Excedrin*'s ingredients is aspirin—250 mg of it. Another is acetaminophen (250 mg), an analgesic roughly com-

parable to aspirin for relieving pain and fever. Acetaminophen's advantage is as an alternative drug for those allergic to
aspirin or for others who should not take aspirin for any of
several reasons (see page 27). CU knows of no such advantage
when acetaminophen is combined with aspirin in *Excedrin* or
other shotgun preparations.

Until the product was reformulated as of June 1980, *Excedrin*'s third ingredient was 129.6 mg of salicylamide. Evidence
shows that the makers of *Excedrin* were not losing much when
they dropped salicylamide. *AMA Drug Evaluations* reports
that salicylamide "is much less effective than aspirin" for pain
or fever when given in the same dose, and that it is "too weak
and unreliable to be useful." Similarly, the FDA advisory panel
reported that studies have shown that salicylamide does not
have any superiority over aspirin in doses below 600 mg and,
indeed, at such low dosage, is indistinguishable from placebo.
It further reported that an average of 2,000 mg of salicylamide
every four to six hours is needed to show a moderate-to-marked
analgesic effect. The panel concluded that salicylamide is ineffective in currently recommended doses of 300 to 600 mg; and
there is insufficient information to determine the safety and
effectiveness of its combination with acetaminophen or aspirin.

Finally, one *Excedrin* still contains 64.8 mg of caffeine,
almost twice as much as *Anacin* or *Bromo Seltzer.* So those
who take eight *Excedrin* tablets in a day—the maximum
recommended on the label—are getting about 518 mg of caffeine, or the equivalent of four cups of coffee. Thus it is not
surprising that some people who take the maximum daily dosage of *Excedrin*—on top of their usual caffeine intake in coffee,
tea, and cola drinks—may become jittery.

With the 1980 reformulation, *Excedrin* is now called a "new
extra-strength pain reliever." Like *Anacin, Excedrin* sells at a
premium. Also like *Anacin, Excedrin* is a costly way to get an

Ingredients of selected analgesic products

Product	Aspirin	Other analgesic
Alka-Seltzer*	324 mg	—
Anacin	400 mg	—
Arthritis Pain Formula	486 mg	—
Arthritis Strength Bufferin	486 mg	—
Bayer Aspirin	325 mg	—
Bayer Timed-Release Aspirin	650 mg	—
Bufferin	324 mg	—
Cope**	421.2 mg	—
Ecotrin	325 mg	—
Empirin †	325 mg	—
Excedrin	250 mg	acetaminophen, 250 mg
Excedrin PM**	—	acetaminophen, 500 mg
Vanquish	227 mg	acetaminophen, 194 mg

*Also contains citric acid (1,000 mg).
**Reformulated to exclude aspirin and the antihistamine methapyrilene, which was banned by the FDA. *Excedrin P.M.* now includes the antihistamine pyrilamine.

Caffeine	Antacid
—	sodium bicarbonate, 1,904 mg
32.5 mg	—
—	aluminum hydroxide; magnesium hydroxide‡
—	aluminum glycinate, 72.9 mg; magnesium carbonate, 97.2 mg
—	—
—	—
—	aluminum glycinate, 48.6 mg; magnesium carbonate, 97.2 mg
32.5 mg	aluminum hydroxide, 25 mg; magnesium hydroxide, 50 mg
—	—
—	—
64.8 mg	—
—	—
33 mg	aluminum hydroxide, 25 mg; magnesium hydroxide, 50 mg

†Product formerly known as *Empirin Compound*, which combined 227 mg of aspirin, 162 mg of phenacetin, and 32.5 mg of caffeine.
‡Quantities not available from manufacturer.

effective dose of pain reliever, plus an ingredient (caffeine) whose rationale in an analgesic is unproved.

Vanquish is merely a further variation on the same familiar theme—but it has *five* ingredients. Like *Excedrin, Vanquish* contains aspirin, acetaminophen, and caffeine; and like *Bufferin,* it includes small amounts of two antacids. *Cope* also contains aspirin and caffeine, plus the same two antacids as *Vanquish. Cope* had a fifth ingredient, the antihistamine methapyrilene, but it has been dropped. The same antihistamine no longer in *Cope*'s formulation was also formerly found in *Excedrin P.M.*

In April 1979 the National Cancer Institute (NCI) reported that methapyrilene causes liver cancer in rats and mice and should be presumed to do so in humans. The FDA reached the same conclusion after evaluating the NCI's data. Wasting no time, the FDA in June 1979 recalled most of the OTC drugs containing methapyrilene. The announcement was made jointly by Joseph A. Califano, Jr., then secretary of Health, Education, and Welfare (HEW), and the Proprietary Association (whose members make 80 to 90 percent of the nonprescription products containing methapyrilene). Califano said: "This substance poses a potential risk to humans. . . . Consumers should consult the ingredients list on medicine in their possession to see whether methapyrilene appears." Among the OTC products involved in the recall besides *Cope* and *Excedrin P.M.* were *Compoz, Nytol, SleepEze,* and *Sominex.*

Taking note of the proliferation of ingredients in analgesics, the FDA advisory panel on internal analgesics said that, in general, the fewer ingredients in OTC products, the safer and more rational the therapy. Yet the panel endorsed combination products, although recommending that "no more than two safe and effective analgesics" be permitted in one product. CU's medical consultants disagree with this endorsement even for two-ingredient combination products. They know of no studies that show the superiority—milligram for milligram—of a two-drug analgesic combination over a single-ingredient product. What's more, a combination product exposes an individual to the toxicity and allergic potential of two ingredients. CU urges FDA Commissioner Jere Goyan to restrict analgesic-containing products to no more than one safe and effective analgesic component.

The American Pharmaceutical Association has also taken a stand against combination drugs. Its *Handbook of Nonprescription Drugs* advises: "Recent claims promoting 'extra-strength pain relievers' require clarification. Such products are usually combinations of several analgesic ingredients and may include acetaminophen, salicylamide, and aspirin. Because the total analgesic ingredients may be more than 325 mg, or 5 gr, the implication in these products' promotional materials is that they are 'stronger' and hence more effective. These claims only confuse the consumer because combinations have not been proven more effective than the sum of their individual ingredients. In most controlled clinical trials, pain relief provided by analgesic combinations has not been superior to that of aspirin alone."

There is no doubt about the effectiveness of aspirin. Many drugs are greeted with great enthusiasm when first marketed; subsequent experience tempers the initial glow. But aspirin is different. Well-controlled studies suggest that it is even more effective than was once supposed.

A Mayo Clinic study published in 1972, for example, compared plain aspirin not only with acetaminophen and phenacetin, but also with a range of allegedly more potent and far more expensive pain relievers available only on prescription—including codeine, propoxyphene (Darvon), ethoheptazine (Zactane), and mefenamic acid (Ponstel). Each drug was given orally, in random order. The dosage for each was the recognized therapeutic equivalent of that for the other drugs, and all were enclosed in identical blue capsules. Some capsules were placebos. The tests were double-blind; that is, neither physicians nor patients knew what the capsules contained until the results were recorded. The fifty-seven patients in the study all suffered from pain judged to be mild to moderate, occurring in various parts of the body and associated with inoperable cancer.

The results can be summarized briefly. No drug in the study had a significantly faster onset of relief than aspirin or a significantly longer duration of relief than aspirin. The number of side effects reported for aspirin did not differ significantly from the number reported for the placebo. Aspirin led the list when it came to the number of patients experiencing at least 50 percent relief of pain. The average estimated percentage of pain relieved was higher for aspirin than for any other drugs.

The investigators concluded: "In this study, simple aspirin at a dosage of 650 milligrams [equivalent to two 5-grain tablets] was the superior agent for relief of cancer pain among the tested marketed analgesics. Indeed, among all analgesics and narcotics available for oral use, none have been demonstrated to show a consistent advantage over aspirin for the relief of any type of pain."

An interesting but not unexpected sidelight of the study was the response of patients to the placebo. Twenty-one percent claimed greater than 50 percent relief of pain with the dummy medication. Such a result, which is common in medical experience, is called the placebo effect. In essence, many of those who believe a certain medication will help them obtain relief from it even if it has no known pharmacological effect. The same principle often applies to OTC remedies, and sometimes explains why one drug seems to work while a virtually identical one does not.

Moreover, Darvon, one of the expensive prescription analgesics used in the Mayo Clinic study, had been shown in an earlier study published in *The Journal of the American Medical Association* to be no more, and perhaps less, effective than aspirin. The authors of the report noted, "The fact that a drug is sold by prescription in no way proves its efficacy and potency." They concluded: "Our review prompts us to recommend aspirin as the mild analgesic of choice. If aspirin does not provide adequate relief, it is unlikely that Darvon will do so." The safety of Darvon has been questioned. Its potential for abuse has been noted by some physicians and it has also been implicated in deaths from drug overdose. In June 1979, Califano, then HEW secretary, requested the surgeon general of the United States, Julius Richmond, to coordinate studies of the drug and to report the results within a year, if possible. Meanwhile, Eli Lilly & Co., the makers of Darvon, agreed in July 1979 to distribute voluntarily to physicians a warning telling of the hazards of using the drug in excess or in combination with other drugs or with alcohol. This circular was called inadequate by Califano just prior to his departure from the HEW post.

For people who are allergic to aspirin, have stomach disorders, gout, bleeding tendencies, or are taking anticoagulants, antidiabetic or arthritis drugs, CU's medical consultants recommend acetaminophen. Most studies indicate that in similar doses acetaminophen is roughly comparable to aspirin in reducing fever and for relief of various common aches and pains. Because it lacks aspirin's effect on inflammation, however, acetaminophen cannot replace aspirin in the overall treatment of connective tissue diseases such as rheumatoid arthritis during the acute flare-up stage. Advantages of acetaminophen, however, are many: It can be used by people who are allergic to aspirin (although there may be allergy to acetaminophen); it doesn't cause stomach bleeding or affect blood clotting; and, unlike aspirin, it is stable in liquid preparations, a useful dosage form for children and others who may have difficulty swallowing tablets. Acetaminophen can be purchased without a prescription under its generic name and under ten or more brand names—such as *Liquiprin* (for children), *Tempra, Tylenol,* and *Valadol.* As in the case of aspirin, CU recommends buying the least expensive brand.

The dosage schedule for acetaminophen is identical to that for aspirin (see page 30). The FDA advisory panel recommended that acetaminophen labels warn consumers not to exceed the recommended dosage because large doses can cause

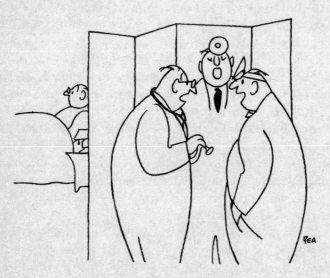

"Aspirin!" "Aspirin!" "Aspirin!"

death from irreversible liver damage. The panel also reported that there is no basis for the claim that acetaminophen is safer than aspirin, an impression conveyed by some acetaminophen advertising.

Although *Alka-Seltzer* is widely advertised as an antacid for digestive disturbances, CU's medical consultants advise against its regular use for that purpose because its aspirin content makes it unsuitable as a digestive aid (see Chapter 7). As a pain reliever, though, *Alka-Seltzer* has some merit. It must be dissolved in a glass of water before it can be taken, which reduces its time in the stomach, hence minimizing possible gastric irritation. However, it contains so much bicarbonate that it should *not* be taken daily over long periods. And its sodium content is so high that it should not be used *at all* by anyone on a low-salt diet, as the current label warns. Those tempted by the ads to depend on *Alka-Seltzer* for regular relief from the simultaneous discomfort of headache and upset stomach should take particular note of such warnings against the frequent use of *Alka-Seltzer*.

An *Alka-Seltzer* tablet contains 324 mg of aspirin. For relief of mild to moderate pain, two *Alka-Seltzer* tablets, therefore, are about equivalent to two aspirin tablets. The cost, of course, is substantially higher. Because of its high price and sodium bicarbonate content, CU's medical consultants do not recommend *Alka-Seltzer* (or a similar product such as *Fizrin*) over plain aspirin taken with a full glass of water. However, for a person who experiences mild stomach distress even when aspirin is taken with the recommended quantity of water, the occasional use of a soluble form of aspirin would seem to be reasonable.

Aspirin's caveats are important.

- Prolonged use of aspirin for chronic conditions, such as rheumatoid arthritis, should be monitored by a physician. The

FDA panel's recommendation for the label warning on aspirin and all analgesic products states: "Do not take this product for more than 10 days. If symptoms persist, or new ones occur, consult your physician."*

- Drink a full glass of water or other liquid with aspirin to minimize possible stomach irritation. If you experience mild stomach distress when you take aspirin, consider acetaminophen or a soluble form of aspirin, which can be dissolved in a glass of water before you take it.

- The FDA advisory panel recommended that the standard dosage for aspirin and acetaminophen be 325 mg or 5 grains per tablet. And if a tablet does not contain the standard dosage, it must be clearly labeled "non-standard."

- Unless instructed to do so by your physician, do not take more than 10 to 15 grains (two or three tablets) at a time, do not take aspirin more often than every four hours, and do not take more than ten tablets in twenty-four hours. One of the earliest symptoms of chronic aspirin overdosage is ringing in the ears, sometimes accompanied by a decrease in hearing ability. These effects are reversible when the dosage is lowered.

- Some people are sensitive or allergic to aspirin (shortness of breath and wheezing, skin rash, hives). If you are among them, acetaminophen is a reasonable alternative. Since a wide variety of combination OTC products contain aspirin, be sure to read labels. The panel's recommended label warning states: "This product contains aspirin. Do not take this product if you are allergic to aspirin or if you have asthma

*The antirheumatic properties of aspirin have been purposely omitted by the panel in its consideration of safety and efficacy. The diagnosis and treatment of rheumatic diseases should be left to a physician and should not constitute any part of a label claim for aspirin.

except under the advice and supervision of a physician."

- Patients with a history of stomach ulcers or gout as well as those on oral antidiabetic medications should consult a physician before taking aspirin. The panel's recommended label warning for such patients is: "Caution: Do not take this product if you have stomach distress, ulcers or bleeding problems except under the advice and supervision of a physician."

- Aspirin retards blood clotting in several ways. Hence patients with bleeding disorders and patients using anticoagulants such as warfarin (Athrombin-K, Coumadin, Panwarfin) should take aspirin sparingly, if at all. There is also some evidence that pregnant women (see Chapter 22) should not take aspirin during the last three months of pregnancy because of possibly affecting the blood-clotting mechanism of the newborn. Among pregnant women taking high dosages of aspirin there is some evidence of added risk of prolonged labor and an increase in the average duration of pregnancy.

- Patients due to undergo elective surgery should not take aspirin one to two weeks before they are scheduled for hospitalization because of aspirin's effect on blood clotting.

- Keep in mind that aspirin and alcohol are not a safe combination. Since each of these drugs is an irritant to the stomach lining, CU's medical consultants warn that combining the two (e.g., treating a hangover with aspirin) may increase the risk of gastrointestinal bleeding from either drug. As for acetaminophen, it may have its potential for liver toxicity enhanced when taken by chronic alcoholics who have liver disease.

- For children's doses, consult the label. The dosage for children recommended by the FDA is on page 32. Children can be given the recommended dose crushed in a little applesauce or honey if they dislike taking it straight. If children prefer to take their aspirin adult-style, be sure they drink a full glass of liquid along with it. CU's medical consultants warn against keeping flavored aspirin in the home because a child could mistake it for candy.

- Keep aspirin and other drugs out of reach of children. In 1976, the latest year for which statistics are available, twenty-five children under five years of age died after ingesting overdoses of aspirin or other salicylates. This total accounted for about 21 percent of all accidental deaths from poisoning among children in that age group. However, the

Recommended aspirin dosage schedule for children

The following table lists the number of aspirin tablets that children ages two through eleven can safely take every four hours. (Parents should not administer aspirin to a child less than two years old except with the advice and supervision of a physician.) No more than five single dosages of aspirin should be taken in a twenty-four-hour period. Nor should aspirin be taken for more than five consecutive days except with the advice and supervision of a physician. Children's tablets are 80 mg or 1.23 grains each; a standard adult tablet is 325 mg or 5 grains.

| Age | Number of tablets that can be taken every 4 hours | |
	Children's tablets	Standard adult tablets
2 to under 4	2 (160 mg)	½ (162.5 mg)
4 to under 6	3 (240 mg)	¾ (243.8 mg)
6 to under 9	4 (320 mg)	1 (325 mg)
9 to under 11	5 (400 mg)	1¼ (406.3 mg)
11 to under 12	6 (480 mg)	1½ (487.5 mg)

number of children under the age of five years who were hospitalized for longer than one day as the result of aspirin or salicylate ingestion has decreased from 373 in 1973 to 168 in 1976 mainly as a result of the 1972 law on poison prevention packaging.

- The use of so-called timed-release aspirin preparations is not advised. As with so many of these products, absorption may be irregular and adverse reactions prolonged.

Finally, CU's medical consultants have two basic recommendations.

First, question all claims made for OTC analgesics—indeed for all OTC drug products. Do not wait for FTC challenges to be skeptical of these claims. Encourage your children and your friends to be skeptical of all such advertising, too. The FDA panels on OTC drugs, in addition to creating standards for safety and efficacy, are also making recommendations for label claims in order to eliminate ambiguity and puffery. But until implementation is completed, don't be taken in.

Second, when selecting an analgesic, limit your consideration to the cheapest available brand of plain aspirin,* or if a substitute is required, the cheapest available brand of acetaminophen.

---

*In Canada "aspirin" is still a Bayer trade name, so other brands of aspirin are identified by the generic name acetylsalicylic acid, or ASA.

2
Colds and coughs

Since the discovery of penicillin in 1928 there has been more progress toward the prevention and treatment of infectious diseases than in all the rest of medical history combined. Smallpox has now been eradicated, typhoid fever has become a rarity, and pneumococcal pneumonia is both curable and, now, preventable. And yet no means has been found, to date, to eliminate or cure the common cold, which, it has been estimated, costs $5 billion each year in lost wages and medical expenses.

In fact, the common cold is not a simple matter; rather, it is a complex of symptoms. Caused by any one of a group of viruses (more than 120 different viral strains that produce common cold symptoms in humans have been isolated), the common cold is primarily an infection of the lining membrane of the upper respiratory tract, including the nose, the sinuses, and the throat. This delicate membrane reacts to infection by swelling and by increasing its rate of mucus formation, leading to congestion, stuffiness, and a great deal of nose blowing. Due to loss of the nasal cavity as a resonating chamber, a characteristic change in voice quality also occurs. The increased mucus flow usually causes a postnasal drip, which is irritating and contributes to the familiar "scratchy" throat and cough.

The sinuses, which normally empty into the nasal cavity, may become blocked by excessive swelling of the membranes. The resultant increase in sinus pressure may cause a headache. In similar fashion, swelling in the upper part of the throat can block the Eustachian tubes—the two narrow canals that lead to the ears. This blockage can cause accumulation of fluid and pressure in the middle ear, which may be painful. Less commonly, an unpleasant spinning sensation known as vertigo may result.

A cold is usually self-limited, lasting about one to two weeks. At any time during the course of a cold, bacteria (such as staphylococci or pneumococci) can be secondary invaders, bringing on painful infections of the sinuses and ears. However, the old warning that, if you don't take care, a cold will turn into pneumonia, is hardly ever true. Pneumonia and most other infections of the lower respiratory tract begin in the bronchi and the lungs rather than in the upper respiratory tract.

Most people stay home from work or school because of generalized symptoms—muscle aches, weakness, and fatigue. The extent of these symptoms varies from person to person. Although mild elevation of temperature can occur with the common cold, a rectal temperature above 101°F is usually a sign of a more serious viral or bacterial infection. If fever above 101°F, taken rectally, persists beyond two days, medical advice should be sought.

Americans spend more than $900 million a year for cold and cough remedies. Advertisers have claimed preventive and curative virtues for vitamins, alkalizers, lemon drinks, antihistamines, decongestants, timed-release capsules, antibiotics, antiseptic gargles, bioflavonoids, nose drops and sprays, quinine pills, aspirin mixtures, laxatives, inhalers, aromatic salves, liniments, room air sprays, and a variety of other products. There are at least 300 over-the-counter (OTC) products—most of which are a combination of ingredients—marketed for the treatment of symptoms of the common cold. Many of these drugs do neither good nor harm to the cold victim—but there is no doubt that they benefit the drug manufacturers.

Everyone has heard of sure-fire formulas for preventing a cold. Popular home methods include a cold shower, regular exercise, and a hot rum toddy. Some people swear by cod-liver oil, tea with honey, citrus fruit juices (or massive doses of vitamin C), or keeping one's feet dry. At one time, many large firms encouraged their employees to submit to inoculations with cold "vaccines." And splendid results from these programs were regularly reported. But such vaccines, like many other "scientific" (or folk) remedies, gradually have been abandoned as experience and controlled testing have proved their uselessness in preventing colds. Now, just as fifty years ago, Americans on the average will suffer two to three colds a year, the acute infectious stages of which will last about a week or two (although a cough or postnasal drip may linger), regardless of any physical measure, diet, or drug used to try to head off the colds. U.S. Public Health Service (PHS) studies show that, during the winter quarter of the year, 50 percent of the population experiences a common cold; during the summer quarter, the figure drops to 20 percent.

It is unfortunate that the name "cold" has been given to this common, but minor, malady. The name has led many people to infer that the common cold is somehow caused by walking bareheaded in the rain, not wearing enough winter clothing, or getting caught in a draft. There is as yet no evidence that the common cold ever occurs in the absence of an infecting organism. Moreover, studies have shown that chilling does not predispose one to infection with the cold virus (or viruses). The increased incidence of colds in winter reflects the fact that people spend more time indoors, thereby facilitating the transfer of viruses from person to person. In fact, one is less likely to catch a cold after exposure to the elements than after mixing with a convivial group of snifflers and sneezers at a fireside gathering.

The common cold, it is now reasonably certain, is not only spread by sneezing and coughing but also by shaking hands and handling contaminated articles. The home, office, classroom, bus, or any other place where people gather is a good spreading ground. But resistance seems to vary greatly among individuals, so that not everyone exposed to a common source of infection becomes ill. Moreover, the natural factors—whatever they are —that contribute to resistance in an individual may be operative at one time and not at another. Thus it is not uncommon for some unlucky person to have a "bad year," suffering from as many as five or six colds, and then remain in excellent health during the following year or two. These variations in resistance and the irregular pattern in the occurrence of colds make it extremely difficult to evaluate the effect of any medication on the course of the common cold.

This has not stopped the manufacturers of cold preparations from palming off on an all-too-willing public a series of gimmicks and "cure-alls" for the prevention or treatment of cold symptoms.

Because one way colds are transmitted is by small moisture droplets in the air, attempts have been made to sterilize the air —with special ultraviolet lamps, with sprays of chemicals such as triethylene glycol, or with air purifiers containing "germicidal filters" or producing negative ions. These attempts have not been successful.

Another attempt at sterilizing the air involved medication delivered by means of aerosol spray. The product released a mist compounded of menthol (an organic alcohol with a medicinal scent), glycols (antibacterial agents long ago shown to be without therapeutic value when sprayed in the air), and flavoring oils. Even if the ingredients were effective, common sense should make one wonder how a large enough dose could be delivered when the product is so widely dispersed in the air. Furthermore, Consumers Union's medical consultants do not know of any published reports of controlled trials supporting the claim that these preparations can relieve congestion.

After the death of a five-year-old girl who had been exposed to *Pertussin Night-Time Medicated Vaporizer Spray,* the Food and Drug Administration (FDA) in 1973 ordered the recall of that preparation and later reported that twenty-one deaths since 1968 had been associated with its use. The FDA attributed the spray's toxicity to the presence of trichloroethane, an organic solvent. Five additional brands having the same chemical solvent as an ingredient in the spray were also recalled by the FDA. An advisory panel of health professionals reporting to the FDA in 1976 stated that, on the whole, aerosol decongestant sprays have been generally safe when used as directed, but that there have been reports of deaths from deliberate abuse that cannot be overlooked. The panel concluded that, although aerosol products do possess inherent advantages for specialized application of drugs in bronchial asthma and other acute respiratory conditions, the possibility of toxic effects of the halocarbon propellants should be carefully evaluated by a suitable panel of experts in this area.

Most medical scientists now agree that until an antiviral drug is developed, or until a reliable cold vaccine is perfected, no real progress in limiting the spread or incidence of colds can be anticipated. But if colds can't be prevented, can the symptoms at least be checked or relieved? Here, too, there are determined advocates of a wide variety of home remedies and equally determined supporters of the large number of OTC products. One reason why much research on cold remedies is scientifically worthless is because of the difficulty in making an accurate diagnosis of the common cold. The term "cold" has been applied not only to viral respiratory infections but also to almost any one of a variety of factors that cause congestion of the nose, including irritants, smog, or allergens. Such noninfectious congestion may last a few minutes, several hours, or even a few days. Any medication, even a placebo, may seem to be remarkably effective especially if the congestion is of short duration. Studies have also failed because they did not allow for the unpredictable course of colds and their varying incidence. Emotions may also play some part in the variability of the common cold.

In 1970 interest in vitamin C was revived by Linus Pauling, Ph.D., with the publication of his book *Vitamin C and the Common Cold.* Pauling cited several experimental studies, anecdotal evidence, and personal experience to support his belief that large doses of vitamin C can prevent or cure the common cold and possibly other respiratory infections as well.

After careful scrutiny and thoughtful consideration, *The Medical Letter* and CU's medical consultants and statisticians judged that the studies cited were inadequately controlled. Differences in individual resistance and the natural course of an untreated respiratory infection, *The Medical Letter* noted, have an important bearing on the apparent effects of any proposed remedy. Thus a well-designed, controlled trial that is double-blind must be conducted over a sufficiently long period and must include hundreds of persons to give meaningful results.

The first well-controlled study of vitamin C and colds was published in Canada in 1972. More than 800 people were involved in the double-blind study, which extended over several months. There were no statistically significant differences in the number or duration of colds between the vitamin C group and the placebo group. The study did show, however, a significant reduction in the total number of days (1.04 days per cold for the vitamin C group versus 1.32 days per cold for the placebo group) lost from their jobs by the vitamin C group, because their illness was characterized by a "lower incidence of constitutional symptoms such as chills and severe malaise." A subsequent study by the Canadian researchers obtained similar results but failed to show any advantages of large doses of vitamin C over smaller doses. (See "Is Vitamin C Really Good for Colds?" *Consumer Reports*, February 1976.) Well-controlled studies in 1976 and 1979 similarly failed to show any beneficial effect of vitamin C in the prevention or treatment of colds.

A 1973 editorial in the *British Medical Journal* said about vitamin C that " too little is known about the possible harmful effects of taking too much." While vitamin C has been promoted as "essentially nontoxic" and "harmless," CU's medical consultants are not so sure, particularly in view of the extremely large doses recommended in Pauling's book (over 300 times the recommended daily allowances now set by the Food and Nutrition Board of the National Research Council). Diarrhea to the point of being disabling can result from excessive doses of vitamin C. Some people, the pregnant and the elderly, for example, and those with certain illnesses—diagnosed or undiagnosed—might run even greater risks than the medically "normal" person.

Chronic urinary acidification, which is likely with a daily ingestion of 4 grams or more of vitamin C for a period of months, may increase the frequency of kidney stones in persons with gout. And ingestion of 10 grams of vitamin C a day for several days might, in the judgment of some authorities, impose a formidable acid load on the body, especially for people with impaired kidney function. Also, large amounts of ascorbic acid in the urine interferes with urine sugar testing. Two popular methods currently employed by diabetics involve color reactions following the testing of urine with a tablet or paper tape. With the tablet *(Clinitest)* method, ascorbic acid can alter the color reaction and give an erroneous impression of excessive sugar in the urine. Diabetics who use *Testape* (a paper dip method) and take high doses of vitamin C may be falsely reassured because ascorbic acid interferes with the color reaction indicating sugar in the urine. Either of these incorrect results could thus cause some diabetics to change their medication dosage, with possibly serious consequences.

In addition, some authorities suspect that excessive vitamin C during pregnancy may result in infants who, despite normal intake of vitamin C after birth, may develop scurvy because their enzyme system had adjusted to high levels during the fetal period. Finally, the fad for vitamin C has led some persons to use a version of it containing sodium ascorbate, which could carry a special hazard for those on a low-sodium diet.

There is some evidence, on the basis of experiments with animals, to suggest that large doses of ascorbic acid may have detrimental effects on young developing bones. There are as yet no controlled studies to confirm this possibility in human beings who have been exposed to large doses of ascorbic acid over long periods of time.

Determining the extent of possible dangers (real and theoretical) accompanying a sustained large intake of vitamin C— 250 to 15,000 milligrams (mg) daily over several months—calls for more extensive and better-controlled toxicity studies than are now available. Whatever the purported merits of increasing vitamin C allowances, toxicity studies should precede any efforts to encourage people to take large amounts of any substance, however seemingly innocuous. According to the FDA advisory panel on coughs and colds, labels claiming that vitamins—alone or in combination with other products—are effective as cold preventives or cures should not be permitted. Manufacturers should be allowed to use vitamin C in their products if they so wish for a period of three years, the panel reported. Appropriate studies to document vitamin C effectiveness must be completed within that time period if vitamin C is to be retained in OTC cold preparations. Furthermore, no claims should be made for effectiveness of vitamin C until proof is at hand, the panel said.

The popularity of antihistamines in cold treatment began with an enthusiastic clinical study by a physician who, impressed by the effect of antihistamines on hay fever (an allergy), tried them on people with colds and found them helpful in shortening the colds or controlling the symptoms. Other doctors, impressed by the first report, gave antihistamines to their patients and reported equally favorable results in treating the common cold.

But physicians who are expert clinicians and adept in diagnosis and treatment of illness may not be equally knowledgeable in the careful planning and evaluation of drug trials. Rigid criteria must be met to prove the efficacy of an agent claimed to prevent or treat a disease. When the effect of antihistamines on the common cold was properly investigated, it was found that a placebo gave results just as good as those from the much-hailed drug. In short, antihistamines have proved of no significant value against the common cold; furthermore, even though they do tend to dry the mucous membrane, side effects such as drowsiness, dizziness, and headache make them difficult for many people to tolerate.

The pitch for bioflavonoids for relief of colds came after the disillusionment with antihistamines. Bioflavonoids, a group of complex organic chemicals, are believed—although never proved—to have a strengthening effect on the capillary blood vessels. That bioflavonoids were as disappointing as antihistamines in the treatment of colds also has been amply demonstrated. In 1968 the FDA determined from its findings—in combination with those findings of the National Academy of Sciences–National Research Council—that flavonoid drugs, including bioflavonoids, were not effective "for use in man for any condition." Remedies containing bioflavonoids are no longer widely marketed.

The next fad in the hotly competitive cold remedy field was the introduction of products for oral use containing several ingredients in fixed combinations. (*Contac, Dristan,* and *Ny-Quil* are among the most extensively advertised of this group.) These shotgun preparations contain in varying amounts and combinations a vasoconstrictor decongestant (phenylephrine, phenylpropanolamine, or pseudoephedrine), an antihistamine (chlorpheniramine or brompheniramine), an analgesic (aspirin or acetaminophen), a stimulant (caffeine), as well as vitamin C (ascorbic acid) and other ingredients. The medical profession has consistently repudiated this shotgun approach to medication, but has made little headway against the tide of publicity generated by the pharmaceutical industry.

CU's medical consultants have repeatedly stated that there are few categories of disease for which the use of a fixed combination is warranted—and the common cold is certainly not one of these. Most fixed component formulations force the patient to take unnecessary medications. For example, the inclusion of antihistamines in a cold preparation is irrational, in the opinion of CU's medical consultants. As noted earlier, antihistamines have not been shown to be of value in the treatment of the common cold. Their inclusion in cold capsules "just on the chance that an allergy might be present" cannot be justified, especially in view of the major side effect—drowsiness—associated with their use. Drinking alcohol and taking tranquilizers can magnify these side effects. Antihistamines in cold capsules very likely contribute to automobile and industrial accidents.

Aspirin (or some other analgesic or antipyretic) is often useful for a cold, but is not invariably required by all cold sufferers. Even though aches and pains do accompany a common cold—and a mild fever also on rare occasions—aspirin must be taken in sufficient dosage to be effective. And some cold remedy formulations simply do not include enough aspirin to act effectively either as an analgesic or an antipyretic.

Of all the ingredients in a typical cold tablet, the most rational is the oral decongestant. Most authorities believe that certain oral decongestants—in proper dosage—may help to relieve cold symptoms. Unfortunately, the typical decongestants in most cold remedies work poorly because the dose is too small to do any good. The FDA advisory panel on colds and coughs has helped to remedy this problem by establishing minimal and maximum dosage requirements for those decongestants found to be safe and effective (see page 185).

Among the fixed-combination products, *Dristan Decongestant Tablets* has had a heavy sales pitch. "The exclusive *Dristan* formula cannot be duplicated," claimed the package insert. According to its manufacturer, American Home Products, *Dristan* contained "the decongestant most prescribed by doctors," an "exclusive anti-allergent," and the "pain-relieving medication most recommended by doctors."

What is this remarkable formula? The decongestant is phenylephrine. And doctors do prescribe it often—but to be used as *nose drops,* not orally. Moreover, the oral dose in two *Dristan* tablets (the recommended adult dosage) is only one-fourth of the amount found to be *ineffective* in controlled clinical testing. Also there is a relatively small amount of the antihistamine chlorpheniramine; and like any antihistamine, it is not of much use for cold symptoms.

The pain-reliever "most recommended by doctors" is, of course, aspirin. Each *Dristan* tablet contains the same amount as any 5-grain aspirin tablet. It is therefore true that *Dristan* does "work on aches and fever," as its television ads claimed —but so does any aspirin. *Dristan* also includes a small amount of antacid and about as much caffeine per tablet as 1 ounce of brewed coffee (see page 187). Neither of these ingredients relieves cold symptoms, however. In short, *Dristan* has only one effective aid for a cold: aspirin. But millions of dollars worth of advertising has helped American Home Products sell *Dristan* for roughly twenty times the price of plain aspirin.

Alka-Seltzer Plus Cold Medicine contains much the same type of ingredients as *Dristan:* phenylpropanolamine (a decongestant), chlorpheniramine (an antihistamine), and—aspirin. It is an effervescent tablet that fizzes in a glass of water. But its sole value for cold symptoms is, again, 5 grains of aspirin. Like *Dristan, Alka-Seltzer Plus* sells for much more than unadorned aspirin.

Coricidin D, another shotgun cold tablet, rides the same bandwagon: There is phenylpropanolamine (a decongestant), chlorpheniramine (an antihistamine)—and 5 grains of aspirin. Curiously, the recommended dosage on the label was formerly one tablet rather than two, so an adult who took *Coricidin D* as directed did not even get an effective dose of aspirin. The new dosage now allows for aspirin and decongestant in effective amounts but exposes the cold sufferer to the risk of drowsiness from an unnecessary antihistamine. Unlike *Coricidin D, Coricidin* omits the decongestant.

Since 1971 a new group of products has emerged on television to minister to the sinuses. Such offerings as *Sinarest* and *Sine-Off* have now joined the older *Sinutab* in the war of television commercials against sinus headache and congestion. A look at their label ingredients unmasks these medications as cold preparations in disguise. Each of the three products contains a pain reliever, a decongestant, and an antihistamine. Since sinus headache and congestion are frequent symptoms of a cold, it is not surprising that the same standard remedies are offered. These types of sinus products ring up some $20 million in annual sales.

One of the greatest merchandising successes of all the shotgun cold remedies, *Contac,* came up with a new twist to the formula—the timed-release capsule. But judging by its formula, the people who give their cash to *Contac* are not likely to be helping their colds. In addition to the antihistamine chlorpheniramine, *Contac* contains small amounts of another type of drying agent called belladonna alkaloids. *Contac* also contains 50 mg of the decongestant phenylpropanolamine that can indeed be helpful for a few hours at doses of 25 to 50 mg. Unfortunately, with *Contac*'s timed-release formula, the dosage is theoretically spread out over twelve hours, so the user gets too meager a dose at any one time to be effective against cold symptoms.

Timed-release preparations have been used with dubious success for a variety of prescription drugs as well as OTC cold remedies. In a discussion of such dosage forms several years ago, *The Medical Letter* commented: "Even with the most carefully formulated products, the rate of release in a particular patient is unpredictable. Release may be excessively rapid, or it can take an excessively lengthy period to obtain a sufficient dose of the drug. The widest variation in action must be expected with such medications." The Revision Committee of the U.S. Pharmacopeia (USP) did not recommend timed-release preparations for USP recognition in its 1975 edition because it believes that no such form of any drug has been shown to be essential or valuable in medical practice. CU's medical consultants concur and advise against the use of timed-release preparations. The timed-release formulation is so complex, according to the FDA panel, that it recommended in 1977 that a four-year study be done by the pharmaceutical industry, in cooperation with the FDA, to standardize all OTC timed-release cough and cold products.

CU's medical consultants warn that those who take a multi-ingredient remedy expose themselves to the allergic potential of not just one drug, but of several drugs. The miseries of the cold sufferer could then be compounded by a possible allergic reaction. And when the drugs are formulated into a timed-release preparation, any allergic reaction and accompanying discomfort can be unnecessarily prolonged. Similarly, side effects, which might ordinarily be short-lived, would also be long lasting.

One side effect of oral decongestants, which many people find intolerable, is excessive dryness in the nose, mouth, and throat. This uncomfortable sensation has caused many victims of colds to shy away from these products and simply tolerate their symptoms instead.

A warning is in order for certain cold sufferers who would be well advised to consult their physicians before using any decongestant preparation, either orally or as nose drops. Patients with hypertension (high blood pressure) should be aware that chemicals such as phenylpropanolamine and phenylephrine are "pressor" agents and are thus capable, in sufficient dosage, of raising the blood pressure. Products containing decongestants and caffeine may also cause side effects in patients with thyroid disease and may alter the effect of insulin therapy in diabetics.

Antibiotics, while not useful against colds themselves, are sometimes prescribed by physicians to prevent middle ear infection, sinusitis, bronchitis, or other complications of a common cold. Such dosing may not prevent these complications but might cause complications of its own, including an increase in bacterial resistance or an allergic reaction to the antibiotic itself. Of course, if a bacterial complication does occur—such as otitis (ear infection) or sinusitis—the timely use of an appropriate antibiotic may be helpful. (See Chapter 26 for a discussion of antibiotics.)

The scientists assembled by the FDA to evaluate cold remedies for safety and efficacy expressed their concern over the scarcity of single-ingredient cold products on the market. Almost 90 percent of the cough and cold products they examined contained a combination of ingredients intended to relieve several different symptoms. The panel recommended that combination products for relief of cough and cold symptoms contain no more than four ingredients and called for encouragement of manufacturers to market single-ingredient products. The panel also recommended that such language as "cold medicine," "cold formula," or "for the relief of colds" should be banned from drug labels because it suggests a *cure* when the best the medication can do is to relieve *specific symptoms.*

Meanwhile, the question of what to do for a cold remains. Resting in bed for a day or so, especially if symptoms are severe, may be a good idea for the sake of comfort, but there is no real proof that bed rest shortens the course of the common cold. Taking oneself out of circulation for a day or two may be a good public health measure but has to be balanced against time lost from job or school. To minimize transmission of the cold virus, CU's medical consultants suggest that cold sufferers wash their hands frequently since there is now evidence that the hands may play an important role in virus transfer. Although a handkerchief used for nose blowing is a relatively poor vehicle for spreading the virus, it makes sense to stick to throwaway paper tissues that cut down on the number of times the cold sufferer handles infected materials.

Some authorities endorse familiar folk remedies—chicken soup and aspirin—as being as effective as anything else. Decongestant nose drops or nasal sprays may provide transient relief for a stuffy nose and they might at the same time forestall ear complications by preventing blockage of the Eustachian tubes.

Research has demonstrated that decongestants are more effective when applied topically (as in nose drops) than when taken orally. CU's medical consultants suggest the judicious use of phenylephrine hydrochloride solution USP one-half percent *(Alconefrin, Neo-Synephrine);* one-fourth percent solution is recommended for infants and children. Since nose drops or spray may, after providing initial relief, actually worsen nasal congestion (rebound effect), use of such a product should be restricted to two or three times a day.

For those who can safely use a decongestant (see page 47), and prefer taking an oral one instead of nose drops or spray, the choice among OTC products may be limited. CU's medical consultants know of only two oral decongestants sold as single-ingredient products in effective dosage without a prescription. One is pseudoephedrine *(D-Feda, Novafed, Sudafed);* the other is phenylpropanolamine *(Propadrine).* These medications should be taken only as directed on the label. Phenylpropanolamine is also available in a few combination products that include a pain reliever but no antihistamine. *Ornex, Sine-Aid,* and *Sinutab-II* each offer that combination; some drugstores carry less expensive "house" brands with similar formulas.

Medical advice is rarely required for the common cold. What CU's medical consultants do recommend is patience, since most colds last from one to two weeks whether they are treated or not. Indeed, some authorities believe that any attempt to suppress the symptoms of a cold may actually prolong the infection.

Of all the symptoms that accompany or follow the common cold, cough is perhaps the most irritating. So sought after is relief for "coughs due to colds" that more than 800 OTC cough remedies are to be found on druggists' shelves, and about 100 additional cough mixtures compete for the doctor's prescription pad. With sales of these products so high, it is remarkable that reliable evidence of the effectiveness of most popular cough remedies is virtually impossible to find. Indeed, some studies have indicated that, at least in chronic illness, even the more potent cough-suppressant ingredients used in cough mixtures have no detectable effect at all on the cough itself, although patients treated with these drugs—or with a placebo—*think* they have improved. According to the editors of *The Journal of the American Medical Association,* "Neither practicing physicians nor [the] pharmaceutical industry can produce the objective evidence required under the law on behalf of most cough mixtures."

In fact, the FDA served notice in 1973 that it would ban more than twenty-five brands of fixed-combination cough medicines because of lack of evidence of their efficacy. In 1976 after reviewing the ingredients that go into the myriad of nonprescription cough and cold products, the FDA advisory panel concluded that none of the so-called expectorants was effective and only three basic cough suppressants were both safe and effective (see page 53).

Coughing is a multiple-stage reflex action controlled by a cough center in the brain that responds to irritation in the respiratory tract. Coughing performs an important protective function by both loosening and expectorating secretions, and may even be lifesaving when used to expel a foreign object.

Coughing may also be a nervous act, as in clearing one's throat prior to delivering a speech. A cough can become a disabling ticlike disorder. In other words, coughing is a symptom that may have any one of a number of causes—some innocuous, others serious.

Coughing can usually be relieved by sucking plain hard candies, by drinking hot beverages, or by inhaling steam. Any of these should help limit the frequency and severity of coughing. A cough lingering longer than a week following a cold merits a visit to a physician.

Although tobacco smoke affects people in different ways, heavy smoking unquestionably causes many a cough. Even in a chain smoker, however, it should never be assumed without a thorough medical examination that a cough is caused simply by smoking. The most pernicious aspect of the advertising of cough remedies is that many "smoker's coughs" and "coughs following a cold" may be associated with more serious diseases of the respiratory tract. Such diseases as pneumonia, bronchitis, cancer, or heart failure may be real but unsuspected causes of acute or persistent coughing.

When a cough is caused by an infection, specific therapy can help; in the case of a cough due to pneumonia, for instance, antibiotics can effectively treat the underlying disease in most instances and thereby relieve the cough. One way or another, a cough remedy usually gets into the act, often at the outset and often before the underlying cause of the cough is diagnosed. Although many cough mixtures are relatively ineffective they usually do no harm (in recommended doses): They taste pleasant, and they often have a soothing psychological effect. Coughing patients are prone to demand *something* from their doctors, and doctors often are loath to deny a patient the comfort—psychological or otherwise—of some remedy.

Advertising claims by makers of cough and cold remedies led

to demands by the Federal Trade Commission (FTC) for substantiation. In 1973 the FTC released documents submitted by sixteen manufacturers of thirty-five cough and cold remedies. The public learned, among other things, that *Father John's Medicine* was not—despite wording in ads—prepared according to a doctor's prescription after all, that *Pertussin Plus Night-Time Cold Medicine* "must be used with caution during the day" because of its antihistamine content (which can induce drowsiness), and that *St. Joseph Cough Syrup for Children* —despite its name—does not claim its product is made especially for children.

Most cough mixtures, whether OTC or prescription, are shotgun remedies, containing from two to perhaps ten different drugs aimed at the various links in the cough mechanism. The ingredients can, it is alleged, combat allergies, decrease (or increase) the secretion of mucus, stimulate the sympathetic nervous system, inhibit the parasympathetic nervous system, tranquilize (or stimulate) the patient, depress the cough center in the brain, or depress peripheral nerve reflexes. The theory seems to be that, if you use enough ingredients, at least one should work.

The ingredients with the most obvious effects in typical OTC cough mixtures are sugar and alcohol—the former acting as a demulcent, which seems to relieve sore, irritated mucous membranes, and the latter acting as a central nervous system depressant. Alcohol constitutes 40 percent of *Broncho-Tussin;* 25 percent of *Creo-Terpin* and *NyQuil;* 20 percent of *Cotussis* and *Romilar CF;* and 15 percent of *Trind-DM.* Sugar-free medications are also available for diabetics. *Cerose DM* (Ives), *Codimal* (Central), *Conar Suspension* (Beecham), and *Sorbutuss Syrup* (Dalin) are a few of the sugar-free cough medications identified by the FDA.

The advertisements for *NyQuil* suggest taking the medicine

at bedtime, because it "relieves major cold symptoms for hours to let you get the restful sleep your body needs." Two of the ingredients in *NyQuil* may help to induce sleep—but not by relieving cold symptoms. The alcohol content of *NyQuil* makes the drink 50 proof, and the antihistamine in it (doxylamine succinate) is known to cause drowsiness. Unfortunately, *NyQuil* has too little medication to relieve congestion effectively, and it's often the congestion that hinders sleep for the cold victim. *NyQuil*'s 2.67 mg of ephedrine are far less than the dose usually prescribed for effective decongestant action. Ephedrine is also a central nervous system stimulant, which can work against the product's sedative effect even at that low dosage level.

In September 1976 the FDA advisory panel rated three antitussive (cough suppressant) agents as safe and effective: Codeine, dextromethorphan, and diphenhydramine.

Codeine, a narcotic, is available OTC in combination cough products only in some states. Although codeine is potentially addicting, it rarely causes physical dependence when taken orally for a short time. However, it can cause constipation.

Dextromethorphan acts on the central nervous system (like codeine) and has minimal side effects if taken in recommended doses. It is a nonprescription drug that is safe and effective and should be the drug of choice when an antitussive is indicated, according to the panel. Examples of cough syrups containing dextromethorphan include *Silence Is Golden* (Bristol-Myers), *2/G-DM* (Dow), *Romilar* (Block), and *Triaminicol* (Dorsey).

Diphenhydramine has been used as an antihistamine since 1964, but only recently has its efficacy been recognized as an antitussive. The most common side effect is drowsiness. Diphenhydramine preparations presently are available by prescription only.

Codeine and dextromethorphan, in the amounts present in

cough remedies, can also cause nausea and drowsiness in a significant number of users. And if cough suppressants are taken in doses sufficiently large to suppress the cough reflex, they also may discourage the expectoration or loosening of secretions. This, of course, may not be desirable in some cases of bronchitis or pneumonia. The FDA advisory panel, however, recommended that manufacturers of products containing effective cough suppressants be allowed to make label claims such as "temporary relief of coughs due to minor throat irritation" and "help to quiet the cough reflex." But the labels must advise that the user see a physician if a cough lasts longer than a week following a cold.

In 1973 the FDA published proposed guidelines for the reformulation and relabeling of prescription cough preparations. The FDA cited as its "regulatory philosophy" the belief that medications should include only ingredients of proven effectiveness for the symptomatic relief of common ailments. Accordingly, the FDA stated that it would no longer permit three categories of ingredients in cough preparations. The 1973 guidelines would ban analgesics, such as aspirin and acetaminophen, from these medications and would no longer permit antihistamines and oral decongestants in prescription cough remedies. But the FDA panel in 1976 said combinations that included an antihistamine "for restful sleep" should be allowed to stay on the market for a limited time period, provided testing was undertaken by the manufacturer to establish an effective dose.

The FDA panel, in 1976, found none of the ingredients classified as expectorants to be effective and some to be unsafe. The panel recommended that the following ingredients, whose effectiveness was unproved, no longer be used as expectorants in cough products: Beechwood creosote, benzoin preparations, camphor, eucalyptus oil, menthol, peppermint oil, pine tar, sodium citrate, and turpentine oil. Some ingredients, however, were classified separately pending additional studies to show their effectiveness. In the latter group were ammonium chloride, guaifenesin, syrup of ipecac, and terpin hydrate. Label claims for the group should include "aids in loosening phlegm" or "helps rid passage ways of mucus," but the labels should warn against taking expectorants for persistent chronic coughs.

A vaporizer can help relieve the dry cough that sometimes accompanies a respiratory infection. Its sole job is to humidify the air and loosen secretions in the nose, throat, and trachea. There are two basic types of vaporizers: Electrolytic and cool-mist. There is no difference, therapeutically, in the effect of warm moisture over cool. However, the electrolytic (or steam) type of vaporizer offers some advantages—including more initial relief-giving moisture—but it is not as safe to use as the cool-mist model because of the potential for severe shock. The hazard in using the cool-mist type of vaporizer is in the maintenance of the unit. Special care must be taken to use fresh water each time and to clean the reservoir thoroughly before each use to eliminate the possibility of spraying droplets contaminated with bacteria or fungi into the air. Adding an aromatic product such as *VapoSteam* or *VapoRub* (Vicks) to a steam vaporizer provides very little additional benefit. In a study presented to the American College of Chest Physicians in 1973, laboratory animals exposed to steam vapors of *VapoRub* were reported to experience a decline in their natural defenses against bacterial infection. It is not known whether such an effect would also apply to human beings.

Some physicians favor the use of old-fashioned remedies— mixtures of spirits, honey, and lemon juice, or of hot milk and honey. Medicated lozenges and so-called cough drops are very popular items in the OTC cough-remedy market. In 1978 Americans spent approximately $160 million on this type of cough relief. These products contain varying combinations of benzocaine, honey, camphor, menthol, eucalyptus oil, and flavoring agents—and offer no advantages over less expensive sucking candies, say CU's medical consultants.

For a cough that lasts longer than a week following a cold, a doctor's help should be sought. For chronic coughs, cough remedies and self-medication are not a good idea. There is evidence that the long-continued use of a cough medicine containing a narcotic or one containing a high percentage of alcohol leads to what Henry K. Beecher, M.D., of Harvard Medical School, euphemistically called "an unusual degree of satisfaction in their use." Most doctors, therefore, discourage prolonged use of such remedies for chronic coughs. Some patients, in whom thorough medical investigation has failed to reveal a treatable cause of their coughing, are able to adapt themselves to a chronic cough.

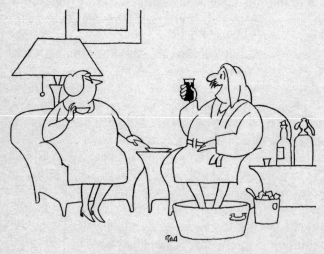

"To the common cold!"

3
Sore throats

A sore throat can be quite uncomfortable. Each swallow of saliva, food, or drink can serve as a cruel reminder. The common postnasal drip, which may be the result of a chronic sinus infection or an allergy, can cause severe throat irritation. In winter some sore throats can be traced to insufficient humidity inside the home. Breathing through the mouth while sleeping can also cause excessive dryness of the mucous membranes. These kinds of sore throats can be avoided by humidification or by eliminating the cause of mouth breathing (by consultation with a physician, if necessary). Dryness of the mucous membranes may predispose one to infections of the upper respiratory tract. In fact, some ear, nose, and throat specialists believe that proper humidification can actually decrease the incidence of throat infection.

The most common cause of a sore throat is infection, and more of these throat infections are viral than are bacterial in origin. However, it is often difficult to tell them apart: Fever, for instance, may characterize both types. Any doubts can usually be resolved by means of a blood count and throat culture, if necessary. The familiar "strep throat" (caused by streptococci bacteria) may sometimes be distinguished by a whitish substance that covers the tonsils. Unfortunately for diagnostic purposes, this appearance can be mimicked by certain viruses, such as the virus that causes infectious mononucleosis.

It is not merely a matter of academic interest to distinguish between viral and bacterial sore throats. If untreated, a strep throat can lead to heart or kidney damage. A ten-day course of penicillin is the treatment of choice for strep throat. (If there is a history of allergy to the drug, other antibiotics are used—see Chapter 26.) Occasionally, other bacteria such as staphylococci or gonococci may cause sore throats, but streptococci account for most bacterial infections.

Viral sore throats are less easy to identify because culture techniques for detecting viruses are much more complicated and are usually not practicable. Some viruses, such as herpes or Coxsackie, often cause small painful ulcerations, commonly called canker sores, on the tongue and in the mouth.

A healthy mouth and throat contain myriads of bacteria and other organisms. The collective name given this germ population is "normal flora." Usually, none of these organisms causes disease. Occasionally, a healthy person may be a carrier of disease-producing bacteria, such as streptococci or staphylococci. When the organism—not readily identifiable in its host's mouth or throat—comes in contact with a susceptible individual, it transfers to the more inviting situation and an infection is initiated. The precise reason why one person is resistant and another vulnerable is not known.

Once bacteria or viruses initiate an infection, the tissues of the throat react to combat it. Blood vessels dilate to increase blood flow to the area, bringing blood cells that act as scavengers. The increased blood flow causes the mucous membranes to redden and the underlying tissues to swell. The swelling is primarily responsible for pain. In a severe sore throat there may be spasms of the throat muscles, which increase discomfort.

Use of antiseptic gargles or medicated lozenges can do little to cure the infection. The offending organisms are deep in the throat tissues, and it is only by means of an appropriate antibiotic in sufficient dosage (taken by mouth or by injection) that adequate amounts of medication can be delivered to the infected area via the bloodstream.

Even less rational is the use of medicated gargles, mouthwashes, or lozenges as sore throat *preventives.* Any antiseptic action of these products is momentary at best, because of the impossibility of sterilizing the oral cavity. The full complement of "normal flora" can be easily restored with the next few breaths, a quick kiss, or even a lick of the lips.

In 1970 the Food and Drug Administration (FDA) served notice that it would no longer permit manufacturers of mouthwashes to claim that their products were of any medicinal value. The agency ordered the manufacturers of eight mouthwashes to cease claiming that mouthwashes could stop bad breath (see Chapter 5), kill germs, or combat colds. The action followed a report prepared for the FDA by the National Academy of Sciences–National Research Council. The mouthwash study found no convincing evidence that mouthwashes have any medicinal advantage over water.

Among the mouthwashes affected by the FDA announcement were *Betadine Mouthwash/Gargle, Cepacol Mouthwash Gargle, Isodine Gargle and Mouthwash,* and *Kasdenol Mouthwash and Gargle.* Mouthwashes were permitted in 1971 to claim "to help provide soothing temporary relief of dryness and minor irritations of the mouth and throat."

One of the biggest-selling mouthwashes, *Listerine Antiseptic,* was not directly affected by the FDA order because it was put on the market before 1938. Congress had strengthened the Food, Drug, and Cosmetic Act in 1962 by requiring manufacturers to prove their claims for the effectiveness of new drugs and all drugs introduced since 1938. But no further clearance was required for older drugs. The FDA, therefore, turned to the Federal Trade Commission (FTC) to monitor advertising claims for *Listerine* and several other pre-1938 mouthwashes on the ground that the mouthwash study's findings were equally applicable to them. As a result, in 1975 the FTC ordered Warner-Lambert Co. to stop advertising that its *Listerine* mouthwash cures or prevents colds or sore throats.

How about the action of gargles against the *pain* of a sore throat? Here the case is not as clear. It is possible that some gargles provide relief from inflammatory pain as a result of an astringent effect on surface congestion or of a transient anesthetic effect, although Consumers Union's medical consultants know of no controlled studies that have tested these possibilities. In fact, the mechanical act of gargling may bring some benefit to the inflamed throat, independent of the specific composition of the gargling solution.

CU's medical consultants recommend warm salt water (one-half teaspoon of table salt to an 8-ounce glass of warm water) both as a gargle and a mouthwash. This mildly concentrated salt solution may help to reduce the painful swelling. In addition, aspirin taken by mouth (but not as a gargle—see page 17) may be helpful in relieving general discomfort. Occasionally, for the pain of a very sore throat a physician may prescribe a mild narcotic such as codeine tablets.

Insistent advertising has pressured many people suffering from a sore throat to swallow some improbable ideas about the efficacy of the gargles, mouthwashes, rinsing solutions, lozenges, and even medicated chewing gum that fill pharmacy and supermarket shelves. One example is the case put forward for *Aspergum.* This chewing gum product is touted as being capable of bringing "fast temporary relief of minor sore throat pain." In fact, topical treatment of sore throats is one of the few tasks aspirin cannot tackle in terms of pain-relief capacity.

The failure of over-the-counter (OTC) sore throat remedies to live up to the implications of their well-hedged claims is one thing; a more serious basis for criticism is the occasional harm they may foster. When people are induced to dose a sore throat with a patent medicine, they may be delaying proper diagnosis and treatment of a potentially serious condition.

As noted earlier, untreated throat infections caused by streptococci can cause heart or kidney damage. Even though many, perhaps most, sore throats are caused by viruses—and not by bacteria—the user of a patent medicine has no way of telling what brought on a particular sore throat. If the sore throat should prove to be viral in origin, the consequences are usually not serious. But the risk involved in not checking into the cause of the sore throat can be serious if the infection should be bacterial and its diagnosis delayed.

Lozenges are also extensively promoted for relief from pain of sore throats. These preparations usually contain a topical anesthetic such as benzocaine. At best, the pain relief obtained from use of a lozenge is short-lived. And any transitory benefits may be offset by the possibility of an allergic reaction to the ingredients in the lozenge.

CU's medical consultants summarize below their recommendations for treating a sore throat.

- Take ordinary aspirin for general discomfort.
- Avoid all other OTC remedies.
- Gargle with warm salt water.
- If the sore throat lasts more than a day or two or is accompanied by fever, check with a physician.

4

Care of
teeth and gums

Loss of teeth need not go hand in hand with aging. But the statistics are not encouraging. Authorities estimate that more than 50 percent of all Americans are toothless by the age of sixty-five. Much of that loss is unnecessary. With the use of available preventive techniques and proper dental care, started soon enough, most people can chew with their own teeth for as long as they live.

Tooth decay and pyorrhea, the most common dental ills leading to loss of teeth, are complex diseases having many aspects that are as yet poorly understood. While both are essentially bacterial diseases, they result typically from an interplay of forces—not necessarily from a specific germ, dietary deficiency, or other single cause. Researchers have not yet precisely determined the importance of each element contributing to the onset, severity, and ultimate outcome of these diseases. The broad outlines, however, are fairly well known.

Tooth decay

Tooth decay (dental caries) is a disease that afflicts at least 95 percent of Americans. The interaction of three factors is chiefly responsible for caries: Bacterial plaque, certain carbohydrates (primarily processed sugar), and an hospitable tooth surface.

Plaque is formed in several stages. The first occurs when a "film" (or pellicle), derived mainly from saliva, develops on the tooth surface. The pellicle becomes full-fledged plaque when it is colonized by streptococci and other bacteria that go to work on sugars and other soluble food residue retained in the mouth. One of the by-products of bacterial activity on sugar is glucan (formerly called dextran), a thick gel-like material that sticks tenaciously to the surface of the teeth and hastens plaque buildup unless it is removed by careful prophylactic measures. Sugar-rich food residue in the mouth is not only the source of glucan; more important, it can be broken down rapidly by bacteria to form acid. Plaque holds the acid against the tooth surface. There the acid attacks the tooth with a success rate that depends on the tooth's vulnerability to decay. The acid forms to a much greater extent in the mouths of people who are highly susceptible to dental decay. The factors responsible for natural resistance to dental decay are largely unknown; one possibility is that they are genetic in origin. Theoretically, anything that prevents production of acid, neutralizes it, removes it quickly from the mouth, or helps the tooth to resist its action should reduce decay.

One approach to the prevention of acid formation is a direct attack on the mouth's streptococcal bacteria. However, some authorities believe that only a small percentage of the total streptococcal bacteria present in the mouth actually accounts for dental decay. Unfortunately, the mouth harbors such enormous numbers of bacteria, and they are so well sheltered by successive overlays of plaque, that it is difficult to immobilize enough bacteria—safely—to reduce acid formation significantly.

Limited success with the antibacterial approach was noted

in studies involving the daily use of an antiseptic mouthwash, chlorhexidine gluconate. The special quality of chlorhexidine gluconate is "substantivity"—the ability to adhere to the tooth surface and to achieve a high concentration at the site of plaque production. When used in a two-year study with Scandinavian students, however, the antiseptic produced disappointing results: Barely significant reduction in plaque and gingivitis (see page 73), and an *increase* in stained, calcified deposits (probably pellicle). Several caries studies with chlorhexidine gluconate also have yielded variable results. About 35 percent of the subjects using a chlorhexidine preparation have shown staining of the teeth as well as of porcelain and plastic filling margins. The ideal substance for the prevention of plaque has not yet been formulated.

Concern has been voiced with regard to chlorhexidine products in which the antiseptic is present in relatively high concentrations (as in skin disinfectants such as *Hibiclens*). The concern is over the mutagenic effect of parachloraniline, which is formed when chlorhexidine is stored. Because chlorhexidine dental products are used at relatively low concentrations (0.2 percent rather than 4 percent as in *Hibiclens*), they *may* not yield enough parachloranaline to be a problem.

The Food and Drug Administration (FDA) has authorized the use of chlorhexidine for clinical tests, but as of September 1979 no applications have been filed with the FDA for dental products containing the drug.

Another avenue of attack on the decay problem involves glucan, the sticky material that helps the bacteria adhere to each other and to the tooth surface. In animal studies an enzyme, glucanase, has been found to break down glucan and reduce the ability of streptococci to generate plaque and cause tooth decay. However, glucanase by itself has not proved effective for human use. An efficacious mixture of enzymes to combat glucan has yet to be formulated.

How about going after the soft, sticky plaque that holds the acid to the teeth? Easier said than done. Plaque differs greatly from person to person. Plaque accumulates constantly, and it seems to do so faster in decay-prone people than in those resistant to caries. Researchers agree that plaque is also the forerunner of calculus (popularly known as tartar), a hard substance that contributes to pyorrhea, a disease of the gums.

The best day-to-day defense against plaque—and food debris as well—is careful attention to oral cleanliness. And you can help by cutting down your intake of sweets not only in amount but also in frequency of ingestion especially between meals. Decay-causing bacteria thrive on candy, soft drinks, cookies, presweetened cereals, and other processed-sugar foods. Acid builds up very fast in the mouth after you eat sweets. People whose teeth decay readily would be wise to stick to fruit and such snacks as celery or carrot sticks for between-meal eating to help reduce exposure to rapid acid formation.

Fluoride can help build a decay-resistant tooth surface when painted onto teeth (so-called topical application). In addition, prophylactic dental paste with fluoride—material reserved by the FDA for the exclusive use of dentists and hygienists to clean teeth—has been shown to reduce tooth decay. Consumers Union's dental and medical consultants strongly recommend multiple use of fluoride:

- Adding fluoride to the water supply or using fluoride supplements during tooth development until the age of twelve.
- By topical application in nonfluoridated areas and even in fluoridated areas if the decay rate warrants it.
- Brushing with a fluoride dentifrice.
- Using a fluoride mouthwash, 0.5 percent daily or 2 percent weekly.
- Using fluoride gel (daily for people with high level of caries).

Self-applied fluoride, dentifrices, mouthwashes, and gels can be used at any age. Adults with gum recession that results in exposed root surfaces are especially vulnerable to root caries and would benefit from self-applied fluoride. Adults who regularly use medications that cause "mouth dryness" or reduced salivary flow should certainly use fluoride.

Fluoride does the best job when it is included in proper amounts in the diet of growing children. As a practical matter, only one way to include fluoride has proved to be highly effective, safe, and inexpensive for large-scale use—fluoridation of a community's water system. Children who drink fluoridated water for the first twelve years of their life average 60 percent less decay than those children who grow up without benefit of fluoride.

Although water fluoridation is the most effective public health measure, self-applied fluoride products such as gels can produce even greater reductions in decay (up to 85 percent). Maximum results can be achieved by combinations such as water fluoridation or fluoride supplements during tooth formation, supplemented with topical and self-applied fluoride after tooth eruption. The actual percentage reductions that can result from different combinations are currently under investigation by the National Caries Program under the auspices of the National Institute of Dental Research.

Evidence, already voluminous, continues to pile up that fluoride in the relatively small amounts needed for decay prevention is safe for people of all ages and for the chronically ill —except for certain kidney patients (see page 68)—as well as for the healthy, and that fluoridation of a community's water supply is by far the best measure now available to bring about a drastic cut in the incidence of tooth decay. Some authorities believe that fluoride may be of limited use in the treatment of osteoporosis, a bone disease occurring frequently in older men and women. In fact, the Food and Nutrition Board of the National Research Council has classified fluoride as "an essential nutrient."

The effectiveness of fluoride against tooth decay is seldom disputed; it is too well documented. Indeed, seven states have legislation requiring municipalities to fluoridate their water supplies. The annual per capita cost of community fluoridation is only a fraction of the cost of filling one tooth. According to a 1978 report in *The New England Journal of Medicine,* community water fluoridation costs only about 10 to 40 cents a year per capita. Despite this fact, community water fluoridation still arouses bitter opposition in certain areas of the United States —some of it based on misunderstandings about the safety of fluoride and some on philosophical objections. Some opponents of fluoridation point to studies purporting to show that fluoride causes a host of ills ranging from mouth ulcers and migraine headaches to mongolism and cancer.* Independent investigations by seven of the leading medical and scientific organizations in the English-speaking world have found no evidence linking fluoridation with cancer. And according to CU's dental and medical consultants, there is no valid evidence for the purported harmful effects of low-level fluoridation.

It is true that fluoride is toxic. But it is toxic only in high concentrations that have no relevance to the amounts taken in by drinking from an optimally fluoridated water supply. Fluoride is often present in natural water supplies, sometimes at relatively high levels. One study compared a community that has a percentage of natural fluoride in its water of 0.4 parts per million with another community that has natural fluoride of 8 parts per million—eight times the 1-part-per-million recom-

*For a report about the attack on fluoridation, see Consumers Union's book *Health Quackery* by the Editors of Consumer Reports Books.

mendation of the U.S. Public Health Service (PHS). By the end of the study, the participants had been exposed to fluoridation for at least twenty-five years. Another study followed the children of two cities, one fluoridated and the other not, for a decade. In both of these and in other studies, no fluoride-related bone abnormalities, pathological effects, or differences in death rate showed up.

Fluoridated water can cause whitish or brownish stains on the teeth of some children. But at the recommended 1-part-per-million level, only a small percentage of children is affected, and the discoloration is usually so slight that it takes a trained eye to detect it. Questions have been raised about the safety of fluoridated tap water for patients with severe or total kidney impairment. Indeed, the National Institute of Arthritis and Metabolic Disease (a division of the PHS) recommends that fluoride—as well as calcium, magnesium, and copper—be removed from tap water *before it is used in an artificial kidney machine.* This recommendation is based on the fact that a kidney patient who needs such dialysis treatment two to three times a week is thereby exposed to about fifty to one hundred times the amount of fluid consumed by the average person. It has no bearing, the PHS says, on the ingestion by *anyone* of optimally fluoridated water from a community water supply.

Nevertheless, CU believes that reports of adverse effects, however isolated and of whatever validity, should not be ignored by the scientific community. For those concerned with public health, there is an obvious responsibility to keep a continuous watch over the effects of such a widespread practice as fluoridation.

Those who oppose community fluoridation on principle, while admitting the value of dietary fluoride, sometimes suggest that individuals who want fluoride could add it to food at home. This would be neither as simple nor as reliable and safe as fluoridation of community water. Although the use of tablets containing fluoride, or its addition to the family drinking water or to fruit juice, has been shown to be an effective procedure, it is certainly more costly and complex. For one thing, a prescription from a doctor or dentist would be required. Since the water in many communities already contains some natural fluoride, each family would have to measure out its own fluoride individually to adapt to the level of fluoride in the local water supply. There would be a problem in making sure that every child obtained enough, but not too much, of the fluoride-bearing food or drink.

The use of tablets containing fluoride obviously poses serious problems not found with community fluoridation. To obtain enough fluoride, children would have to drink all their water at home, or carry fluoridated water when they went out—an impractical regimen to follow. Excessive or prolonged doses of fluoride can be harmful, so parents would have to be careful in preparing the mixture and in storing the tablets out of the reach of children. Tablets taken directly would, of course, require supervision. And for maximum benefit, a family would have to make sure that the tablets (or mixture) were taken faithfully by each child, every single day from birth until at least twelve years of age.

Where water fluoridation is not available on a community-wide basis, another possibility is treatment of the water supply at a local public school by the addition of fluoride at a slightly higher level than usual because the water is used only part time, during school hours. Such procedures have brought a 35 to 40 percent reduction in caries, compared with the incidence in a control group. Fluoride mouthwashes, used weekly under supervision in a double-blind study, have also proved to be effective in reducing caries (by as much as 25 to 30 percent in some cases). Another alternative, one still in the experimental stage, is the possibility of adding fluoride to table salt. A World Health Organization study reported that this technique may prove to be a safe, low-cost, and effective method of fluoridation.

Although fluoride functions most reliably when ingested, children who use water from private wells or live in communities that have not yet begun to fluoridate can receive some benefits from other forms of fluoride application. Even when fluoridated water is used, many dentists recommend that youngsters receive topical applications of fluoride on their teeth until the eruption of the third molar (wisdom tooth). The disadvantage of such topical applications is that they ordinarily must be performed in a dental office or clinic by a dentist or dental hygienist and hence are relatively costly. Such treatments are recommended on at least a yearly basis for those with average teeth; for those with teeth highly susceptible to decay, more frequent treatments may be needed, perhaps continuing until the patients are in their twenties.

Three fluoride compounds commonly used by dentists are fluoride-phosphate, stannous fluoride, and neutral sodium fluoride. Studies have indicated that fluoride-phosphate and stannous fluoride are about equal in efficacy; either may be somewhat more effective than neutral sodium fluoride. Some dentists prefer fluoride-phosphate because the process of application is easier. (New combinations of fluoride and new modes of fluoride delivery are under investigation.)

Fluoride-phosphate can be applied in gel form via a specially made mouth piece that is worn about five minutes a day. Used under supervision for five days a week in a two-year study, this technique resulted in an average reduction of 85 percent fewer caries than in a control group. In an attempt to bypass the complicated and expensive requirement for individually designed pieces, manufacturers have developed preformed pieces in standardized sizes. To adapt to users, these pieces depend on a plastic insert and a viscous gel that adheres closely to the teeth. Whether the procedure will prove as effective with these devices still remains to be determined, along with other questions, such as the optimal frequency for use of self-applied gels.

A less effective method of topical application is the regular use of a special fluoride toothpaste. The American Dental Association (ADA) recognizes six fluoride toothpastes as effective in reducing cavities: *Aim* (Lever Bros.), *Aqua-Fresh* (Beecham), *Colgate MFP, Crest Mint* and *Crest Regular* (Procter & Gamble), and *Macleans Fluoride* (Beecham). People under twenty-five should normally make their choice of toothpaste from this group, since clinical studies have shown their effectiveness. For those who may be sensitive to some of the ingredients in these products, or to their taste, the following additional fluoride toothpastes were judged from CU's 1972 laboratory tests to have some decay-inhibiting potential: *A & P Fluoride, Gleem II,* (Procter & Gamble), *Rexall Fluoride, Safeway Fluoride,* and *Walgreen Stannous Fluoride.*

CU's dental consultants advise all adults to use fluoride toothpaste, but suggest that those with receding gums should first check with their dentists because such pastes might prove too abrasive. Those with rampant caries (and this is a small percentage) and people who risk root caries would be wise to check with their dentists about the supplemental use of a self-applied gel and a fluoride mouthwash, both available by prescription.

A fluoride toothpaste is helpful even when fluoride is available from other sources. Some clinical studies suggest that regular use of a recommended fluoride dentifrice can prolong the effectiveness of a dentist's topical fluoride treatments. In fact, as noted earlier, there are indications that both the use of a fluoride toothpaste and of topical applications are valuable even when fluoridated drinking water is available. CU's dental and medical consultants believe that proper topical applications and fluoride toothbrushing do not increase the body's intake of fluoride beyond recommended limits and do not present any danger of fluoride toxicity to those already drinking fluoridated water. Minute traces of additional fluoride, which might be swallowed with saliva, are not believed to pose any threat to health.

The latest approach to the prevention of tooth decay involves the use of a sealant, a plastic material that is painted onto the biting surfaces of the teeth. The physical barrier thus provided prevents plaque accumulation and the formation of caries. Tests with one variety of sealant showed that for about two years it can be highly effective, resulting in 80 to 90 percent less decay during that period. With longer studies (up to five years), there is an increased tendency for the sealant to be lost with a resulting loss in caries reduction. However, the usefulness of this procedure is largely confined to children, because their biting surfaces are highly susceptible to decay. CU's dental consultants believe the use of sealants may be limited, even for children, because of cost if repeated applications are needed. In states (six so far) where hygienists can apply sealants, it is a more practical procedure. Adults are certainly better off sticking with the standard prophylactic measures and, as soon as decay develops, having their teeth filled with a permanent filling.

Pyorrhea

Even if it were possible to make sure that children entered adult life with decay-free teeth, the battle for dental health would not be over. The other major enemy of teeth is perhaps even more insidious.

Dental decay attacks children and young adults most vigorously. If you're past thirty-five, the teeth you lose will most likely be lost to pyorrhea (periodontal disease). Like tooth decay, pyorrhea is a bacterial plaque disorder. However, it affects not the teeth but the periodontium—the periodontal fiber, gum, and bone that support the teeth. Bleeding and swollen gums are the first warning signs you are likely to notice; irritation—mechanical as well as bacterial—is a frequent cause.

In its early stages, periodontal disease is called gingivitis, and it affects only the gums, or gingiva; if corrected at this time, the disease is reversible.

Pyorrhea virtually always starts with plaque along the gum line. The plaque often becomes mineralized by calcium salts from saliva, thereby forming deposits of calculus. White in the initial stages, these deposits tend to change color to light yellow and then to dark brown, depending on eating and smoking habits and how long the deposits remain in the mouth. They first collect in protected areas around the necks of the teeth, most heavily inside the lower incisors and outside the upper molars—areas near the openings of the salivary gland ducts.

The plaque associated with gum disease is similar to the plaque involved in tooth decay, although it is often thicker and made up of a more complex mixture of bacteria. In the thick plaque associated with pyorrhea, a variety of bacteria produces several noxious products (e.g., toxins and some enzymes), which start a destructive chain reaction in the gums, and in time in the underlying supporting tissues of the teeth as well (see diagram on page 74).

When plaque hardens into calculus, an additional irritant is created: A mechanical irritant affecting the gums every time you chew, swallow, or brush your teeth. Improperly made or overhanging fillings and crowns can have a similar effect. Impacted food residue, retained where the gum meets the tooth, often adds to the abrasive action and increases the irritation.

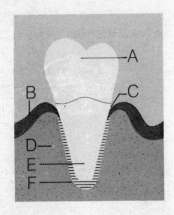 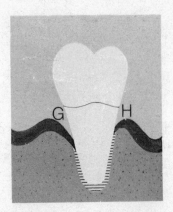

Effects of pyorrhea

Left: A tooth with normal support. Notice that only the crown (A) is exposed. The root (E) is completely enveloped in bone (D) to which it is held by a system of fibers called the periodontal membrane (F). Overlying the bone is the gingiva, or gum tissue (B), which hugs the tooth tightly, leaving only a shallow gingival crevice (C). The tooth at the right shows the effects of damage. The gingival crevice has deepened, and a periodontal pocket (G) has formed. The gingival recession (H) has also exposed parts of the root, and the reduced area of bone support permits the tooth to loosen.

Food also encourages still more bacteria to grow in the plaque, and blood from the gums provides excellent nutrients for the bacteria. The result: Inflammation first, then destruction of gum tissue.

As time passes, the gum tissue separates from the teeth, and a gingival crevice forms and deepens. Plaque and calculus continue to form, extending the bacterial irritation down into the gingival crevice. The healthy, pink gum tissue that normally hugs the tooth and terminates in a fine margin looks swollen, bluish-red, blunted and often becomes tender.

There are more serious consequences. The periodontal

membrane, the system of fibers that connects the tooth's root to the supporting bone, becomes detached. The alveolar bone, the bone that forms the tooth socket, becomes infected and is more and more seriously damaged. Plaque and calculus form ever deeper in the gingival pocket, extending the areas of local infection and inflammation. As increasing amounts of bone are lost from the socket, the tooth has less and less support. The tooth gradually loosens and, unless the process is halted, eventually falls out.

Bad alignment of the teeth may also contribute to pyorrhea. In a well-formed arch, the teeth are arranged evenly and symmetrically, those in the upper jaw meshing properly with the ones in the lower. Adjacent teeth that line up irregularly in the jaw, or teeth in the two opposing jaws that do not contact each other correctly, may set up any of several vicious cycles. They promote retention of dental plaque, since uneven teeth are often hard to clean and their grinding surfaces clean themselves less efficiently than those of properly meshing teeth. They also make it easier for stringy foods such as ham, chicken, or steak to become wedged between the teeth, where they may contribute to chronic gum irritation.

Furthermore, tilted, rotated, or otherwise malposed teeth subject the periodontal structures to abnormal stresses during chewing, which may contribute to a breakdown of the supporting bone. (For that matter, some fairly evenly distributed stresses can also be harmful. Nervous habits—such as frequent clenching of the teeth, lip and cheek biting, and compulsive tongue pressure against the teeth—can contribute to pyorrhea.)

Dental decay that advances far enough to affect tooth position can be a most important factor in pyorrhea. When a tooth is lost to decay, teeth next to the empty space tend to drift toward it. The opposing tooth in the other jaw is also inclined toward the vacant area. In its new position, a tooth that has drifted is inclined, rotated, or extended beyond the level of the adjacent teeth. Spaces between nearby teeth widen, allowing food to collect there and irritate the gums.

If you lose several teeth and don't have them replaced, the remaining teeth may drift so extensively that they no longer function properly. Such a collapse of the entire occlusion produces enough undesirable leverage on the malposed teeth and strain on the supporting structures to affect adversely the supporting bone. The teeth become increasingly mobile, and the destructive forces continue to act on those teeth whose ability to withstand the destruction decreases progressively.

Cigarette smoking, too, is likely to promote gum disease. In 1968 a study of 7,000 people by Roswell Park Memorial Institute, Buffalo, New York, showed that the average periodontal condition of smokers was comparable to that of nonsmokers fifteen years their senior. Dental prospects for young women who smoke were found to be particularly poor; twenty- to thirty-nine-year-old female smokers ran twice as great a risk of being toothless or having advanced gum disease as did nonsmoking women their age. For male smokers, the comparable age range was thirty to fifty-nine.

Systemic diseases, such as diabetes, certain blood disorders, and some nutritional deficiencies increase the tendency of the periodontal tissue to break down. (On many occasions an alert dentist or dental hygienist may note possible signs of early diabetes in a patient, who is then urged to check with a physician.) But since pyorrhea is usually caused by factors in the mouth, a dentist's major effort in therapy is usually to correct the local and more obvious conditions. Special instruments are used to remove calculus from the neck of the tooth and from the periodontal pocket, and then to smooth the tooth root. Any extensively damaged gingival tissue may have to be removed surgically.

After this treatment, the dentist may attack other causative factors. Abnormal occlusion can often be corrected by recontouring areas of the teeth to distribute pressure evenly. Missing teeth should, of course, be replaced promptly by bridgework to prevent drifting. If need be, the teeth in the dental arch can be completely rebuilt. (Even in early childhood, the premature loss of a baby molar deserves attention. A dentist may use space-maintenance techniques to prevent permanent teeth from erupting into faulty positions.)

Brushing and flossing

The major responsibility for the maintenance of healthy teeth and gums and the prevention of periodontal disease and tooth decay lies with the patient—not the dentist. A regimen for continuous plaque control is essential. According to CU's dental consultants, proper brushing and *daily flossing* are needed to prevent the buildup of plaque.

The first rule in dental care is cleanliness. An electric toothbrush can help some people (primarily the handicapped), but CU's dental consultants contend that a powered brush in no way cleans teeth better than a *properly used* manual brush. For those, however, who feel they do a less-than-adequate job of manual brushing and may wish to consider an electric toothbrush, CU recommends that consideration be limited to models approved by the ADA. The ADA's Council on Dental Materials and Devices recognizes those models whose manufacturers have submitted valid clinical evidence that a brush provides "a high degree of oral cleanliness" and does not harm oral tissues.

But for most people the manual brush remains the preferred instrument. And those who wear braces may find electric brushes a nuisance (the bristles may become caught in the wires). In selecting a manual brush, choose a *soft* nylon brush with rounded bristles, one with a head that fits your mouth. There is, of course, a vast number of brushes on the market. The brush design you choose should depend in large part on the brushing technique you use. Therefore, consult with your dentist who can outline an efficient technique for manual brushing and recommend the kind of brush to buy. You may wish to refer to the booklet put out by the American Academy of Periodontology (see page 82) for a good description of a brushing technique. When a soft-bristle brush is used correctly —at least once a day for two to four minutes with proper brushing technique—it will wear out after about six weeks.

With proper brushing and flossing, once-a-day brushing should be sufficient. CU's dental consultants point out that brushing after every meal can't hurt, but that it is probably not necessary if plaque is properly removed once a day. People over twenty-five years old may derive even more benefits from the mechanical action of a properly used brush than from any chemical supplied by a dentifrice. The brushing action removes the mat of plaque (and pellicle, its precursor), which constantly forms on teeth. But in acting against plaque, the brush can be helped by an appropriately formulated dentifrice. To that end, almost all dentifrices contain abrasives and, usually, a soap or detergent. Disclosing agents (tablets or liquids available from the dentist or drugstore), which stain the plaque and highlight areas needing persistent brushing, can be useful.

As a matter of fact, many people do not do a reasonable job of brushing without a dentifrice containing at least some abrasive. If the abrasive is unduly harsh, however, brushers with receded gums are apt to damage the very teeth they are trying to preserve. Exposed root areas are especially sensitive to abrasion. With abrasion, a V-shaped notch is worn into the root of the tooth at the gum line, which weakens the crown of the tooth. For most people, then, *low-to-mild* abrasion is a good thing in regular brushing. But harsh abrasion is never recommended—even for those whose teeth are prone to staining. You are better off with stain than with excessive abrasion; when in doubt, consult your dentist.

The ADA has defined a typical formulation for a dentifrice as containing 20 percent to 40 percent abrasive, 10 percent to 30 percent humectant (a substance that promotes retention of moisture, such as glycerin or sorbitol), 20 percent to 30 percent water, 1 percent to 5 percent thickening agents (carboxymethylcellulose, carrageenan), 1 percent to 2 percent foaming agent, and 1 percent to 5 percent flavoring mixture. With this typical formulation at hand, the ADA in 1977 tested a group of over-the-counter dentifrices for their relative abrasiveness. The association warned, however, that dentifrices can vary from lot to lot, so the results of its test should be interpreted as suggestive and not absolute. Among the toothpastes tested, *Listerine, Craig-Martin,* and *Pepsodent* ranked (in that order) as being low in abrasiveness. Among the products that ranked higher were *Crest, Aim, Phillips,* and *Colgate MFP,* which are listed here in ascending order of abrasiveness.

Toothpastes may have an adverse effect on the gums of a small percentage of people; sensitivity to some elements of a paste's formulation could cause the gums to become shredded or sore. This kind of problem can often be cleared up by switching toothpaste brands. People with gum troubles, those who use an electric toothbrush, and those with fixed plastic crowns should always choose a less abrasive toothpaste such as *Craig-Martin, Listerine,* or *Pepsodent.*

A word now about the cosmetic effects of dentifrices on your teeth: To the degree that ad puffery about "whitening" and "brightening" means anything at all, it seems to relate almost exclusively to the incorporation of one or another of the harsher abrasives into a paste. The ADA has stated that it sees no valid reason for the use of a dentifrice with greater abrasiveness than would be necessary to prevent accumulation of plaque on the teeth.

Some toothpastes have used chloroform for flavoring because of its astringent or "biting" effect. The ADA reported in 1974 that *Ultra-Brite* (Colgate-Palmolive) and *Macleans* still included chloroform; *Close-Up* had dropped the drug from its formulation. After studies showed that chloroform was cancer-causing in animals, the FDA in July 1976 banned the use of chloroform in drug and cosmetic products, including toothpastes. Because the FDA did not also recall existing products, the ban did not affect inventories on the shelves. The ADA reports, however, that chloroform had been removed from both *Macleans* and *Ultra-Brite* several months prior to the FDA's action against the drug. (CU's dental and medical consultants had questioned the need for including such an agent in dentifrices and are gratified that the FDA finally acted to prohibit use of chloroform in toothpastes.)

Ads for *Close-Up, Macleans,* and *Pearl Drops* notwithstanding, none of the dentifrices CU tested contained whitening ingredients, bleaches, or anything else that can in any way alter the natural color of your teeth. You *can* brighten teeth—that is, heighten their luster somewhat—by polishing them. But all the more effective polishers among the tested products were also among the more abrasive. The Federal Trade Commission (FTC) has called on several dentifrice makers to substantiate ad claims dealing with whitening, abrasion, breath-freshening, cavity reduction, and the like. Beecham, for instance, was asked to justify advertising its paste as falling into the lowest third of all pastes in terms of abrasion, a statement CU's study certainly did not support. Beecham having rectified the ads, the FTC reported that no further steps were planned against its advertisements.

Some other special situations deserve comment. Both *Thermodent* and *Sensodyne* have been promoted for "sensitive teeth." But the ADA's Council on Dental Therapeutics reports that it has not seen adequate evidence to justify any such claim. It is worth noting, though, that *Thermodent* was among the least abrasive of the products tested by CU, while *Sensodyne* was not. *Thermodent,* however, contains formaldehyde; CU has questioned its safety in the mouth and stomach. *Extar* has been touted as helpful in removing calculus from teeth and retarding new calculus formation. The ADA, again, was unconvinced.

One recent caution in the selection of toothpastes can now be all but forgotten. In 1972 and 1973 studies reported that most brands of toothpaste contained lead, some in potentially hazardous amounts, in the outer coatings of the tube, in the tube, and in the paste itself. One report stated that of eighteen brands tested only two were completely lead-free. Fortunately, most manufacturers of dentifrices have since switched to non-lead containers and thus have largely eliminated the problem. A representative of the ADA's Council on Dental Therapeutics has reported to CU that it is essentially true that no toothpaste tubes now contain any lead. The FDA also no longer considers the problem to exist. CU's medical and dental consultants have long maintained that all toothpastes packaged in lead-containing tubes should be removed from the market and that the use of lead in toothpaste containers should be prohibited.

Brushing your teeth is only part of a well-rounded program of oral hygiene. A properly used brush can do a good job in removing the bacterial plaque that clings to teeth, but it is apt to miss plaque and food debris nestled in some areas between the teeth. So after you brush, it is important to use dental floss to clean between the teeth.

The American Academy of Periodontology (AAP) recommends the following procedure: Cut off a long piece of floss, waxed or unwaxed, and lightly wrap the ends around your middle fingers. Insert the floss between two teeth and, holding it taut, move it gently back and forth past the point where the teeth contact each other. Move the floss with both fingers up and down five or six times on the side of one tooth, going down to the gum line but not into the gum. Repeat on the side of the adjacent tooth. When the floss becomes frayed or soiled, a turn around one middle finger brings up a fresh section. When you have done all your teeth, rinse vigorously with water (and do that, too, after eating, should you be unable to floss). Some dentists believe that unwaxed floss is better than waxed —CU suggests you ask your dentist for a recommendation. The AAP booklet, "Effective Oral Hygiene," gives suggested techniques for brushing and flossing. It is available for 25 cents from AAP, Room 924, 211 East Chicago Avenue, Chicago, Illinois 60611.

A toothpick is never an adequate alternative to dental floss because it cannot reach into tight areas between teeth. Some dentists, however, suggest a specially shaped toothpick, such as the *Stim-u-dent,* plastic interdental cleaners, or a brush equipped with a rubber interdental tip, because of the possible benefits from stimulation of the gums. If you wish to use a toothpick for removal of material from the mouth, CU's dental consultants recommend that you use it with a special toothpick holder, an inexpensive item available at a drugstore. The holder enables the toothpick to reach many areas of the mouth. Never pick the teeth with wires, pins, or matchbook covers, which can injure the gum between the teeth.

For some of their patients many dentists recommend the use

of a dental irrigator as an adjunct to brushing and flossing. Basically, this device releases a fine stream of water at a fairly high pressure; the user directs the water toward, around, and between the teeth. The idea is to dislodge any food particles and toxic materials that brushing and flossing may not remove. This process can indeed remove some of the irritants present in the mouth, but *not plaque.* Those who use a dental irrigator should direct the stream horizontally, rather than vertically, to avoid forcing debris into gum pockets or under gum flaps. Some dentists believe that at first you should set the pressure low and gradually increase it over days or weeks, instead of starting out with the highest pressure.

Dental irrigators that attach directly to a faucet do basically the same thing as electric irrigators. And faucet irrigators are a lot simpler and less expensive. With no pump and no water reservoir, the faucet models are also more compact than most electric models. Yet they can have their problems too. An adapter must be attached to the faucet, and not all sinks come with faucets that are adaptable. The faucet models cannot be used with separate faucets for hot and cold water and are not recommended for use in homes subject to very high water pressure. A dental irrigator should be considered supplementary to regular oral hygiene. It is *not* a substitute for normal brushing and use of dental floss. However, a dental irrigator could be of particular benefit for those who wear braces or have permanent bridgework. If your dentist has indicated that you should use a dental irrigator, limit your consideration to models that have been judged by the ADA to be safe for unsupervised use. People with poorly controlled diabetes or chronic rheumatic heart disease should consult both their dentist and their physician before using a dental irrigator.

Contrary to much advertising, chewing gum does not provide health benefits to the gums. Hard, fibrous foods (salads and raw fruits) produce a natural cleansing effect, but chewing gum does not. And it can aggravate the stresses and inflammation that go with pyorrhea. Moreover, the sugar in chewing gum—except for the "sugar-free" kind—promotes dental decay.

Dentures and denturism

Of the soak-type denture products CU has tested, *Polident* tablets (or powder) is recommended for maintaining clean dentures. Soiled dentures, however, may benefit from use of *Denalan* or *Kleenite* until the dentures are clean; after that, switch to *Polident.* CU's dental consultants do not recommend the use of plain baking soda for cleansing dentures. And they strongly caution against the use of laundry bleach. Some additional words of advice to denture wearers: If possible, rinse your dentures after every meal; and when you are not wearing them, store them in a cleansing solution (or at least in water —not hot water, urges the ADA).

CU's dental consultants remind denture wearers that regular dental examinations are still essential: Loss of teeth in no way diminishes the need. The dentist will include a check on how the dentures fit and will examine for oral cancer and precancerous lesions.

When a dentist prescribes a prosthetic appliance for a patient, the "laboratory phase" of the process usually is performed outside the office by a laboratory technician. Although the technician actually makes the prosthesis, it is the dentist who works directly with the patient and is responsible for checking the health of the tissues and the proper functioning of the dentures. The dental laboratory technicians who support independent licensure of their occupation so they can be allowed to deal directly with the public are called denturists. Denturism, under the supervision of a dentist, has been legalized in two states: Arizona and Maine. The practice has been legalized in Oregon, to go into effect July 1, 1980—but without the necessity of a dentist's supervision.

In Canada—where the movement originated—organized dentistry had been opposed to the concept but has largely given up the fight because the Dental Mechanics Act is now law. A Canadian study found that prosthetic services provided by denturists are roughly half the price of services provided by licensed dentists. In Canada, before patients can avail themselves of the services of a denturist, they must obtain a "certificate of oral health" from either a dentist or a physician.

In the United States, the ADA has been working hard, both publicly and privately, to fight the legalization of denturism. It is the view of the ADA, and most practicing dentists, that a denturist can provide only a mechanical service, not a full health service. Proponents of denturism claim it reduces prices and extends dental care to older people in need of low-cost dentures.

5
Mouth odor fallacy

Chronic bad breath (halitosis) is a symptom, not a disease. As with many symptoms, there are several possible causes, few of which are more than temporarily affected by *Colgate 100, Lavoris, Listerine,* or other mouthwashes, sprays, drops, tablets, toothpastes, and so on. Most odors are the result of mouth problems—poor oral hygiene, decayed teeth, throat infections, canker sores, pyorrhea (see Chapter 4), postnasal drip, and the like. Such causes are easily detectable, and they need not, if taken care of correctly, result in mouth odors.

The fear of "offending" by means of mouth odor is apparently strong in our society. Many Americans (perhaps those whose "best friends" told them) develop the mouthwash habit. Sales of mouthwashes and gargles amounted to more than $260 million in 1978.

Most people have a disagreeable taste and breath odor upon awakening. This is probably due to bacteria acting on food particles in the mouth during sleep. When a person is awake, bacteria and food particles are regularly dislodged by means of chewing, swallowing, and talking—as well as by random and purposeful tongue movements. During sleep these natural defenses are quiescent. But proper brushing or flossing of the teeth, or dental irrigation, before retiring does much to lessen the likelihood of a "brown" morning taste by removing the debris on which bacteria tend to multiply. The Food and Drug Administration (FDA) advisory panel on over-the-counter mouthwashes, in July 1978, advised that the word "antiseptic" be changed to "antimicrobial" on mouthwash labels and also that such labels refer to *"temporary* reduction in bacteria" because the mouth regains its normal complement of bacteria within a short period of time. Consumers Union's dental consultants suggest that there may be a somewhat greater reduction of plaque if mouthwashes are used to supplement toothbrushing. There have been a number of studies on mouthwashes used as adjuncts to toothbrushing in which the combination appears to be more effective than brushing alone.

Most mouthwashes contain alcohol. Regular use of such products may cause excessive drying of the mucous membranes of the oral cavity and may aggravate preexisting inflammation or infection. CU's medical consultants advise that, if you use a mouthwash, select one without alcohol or one with a minimal alcohol content. Some of the better known brands, together with their alcohol content, are: *Listerine,* 25 percent; *Scope,* 18.5 percent; *Colgate 100,* 15 percent; *Cepacol* and McKesson's *Mouthwash and Gargle,* 14 percent; and *Lavoris,* 5 percent. *Astring-O-Sol* is 70 percent alcohol but its label recommends you dilute "to taste."

The ineffectiveness of commercial mouthwashes in combating halitosis was underlined by an action of the FDA as long ago as 1970. This agency no longer permits manufacturers to claim that mouthwashes have any therapeutic value (see page 59), even in regard to bad breath. Current promotion of these products centers on "freshening" the breath—a temporary effect, at best.

A bad taste in the mouth does not necessarily mean there

is also bad breath. And a person with a sweet mouth taste can have bad breath. A coated tongue may or may not be associated with a bad taste, bad breath, or both. True halitosis occurs most often without changes in the tongue or taste. However, there are some dentists who believe that brushing or cleaning the tongue might possibly help to reduce bad breath.

The pronounced, although temporary, odor that foods containing garlic, onion, and the like give to the breath does not originate in the mouth. It is caused by aromatic material absorbed from the gastrointestinal tract into the bloodstream, carried to the lungs, and then exhaled. Only a small proportion of garlic or onion odor is due to retention of particles in the mouth or between the teeth. Rinsing the mouth may wash away a few particles but will have no effect on the blood level of the odorous substance, which may take many hours to disappear. Smokers may also have a characteristic mouth odor that mouthwashing will not correct.

Mouth spray and drops are also products that impart a pleasing fragrance to the breath—long enough, perhaps, for that good-night kiss, but not for much more. The only possible social benefit to be obtained from mouthwashes, drops, and sprays is the temporary replacement of a bad odor with a nonoffensive aroma. The same is true of the candy mints claimed to freshen the breath by absorbing odors. No substance is known that, in quantities that could be incorporated into a piece of candy, can absorb enough odor to solve permanently the problem of chronic halitosis.

6
"Tired" eyes and eyewashes

Among the heavily promoted over-the-counter (OTC) remedies are the eyewashes, such as *Eye-Gene, Murine,* and *Visine. Eye-Gene* advertises: "Clears red eyes fast. Feel it soothe and refresh tired eyes too." This is a typical eyewash claim.

Although some OTC eyewashes may relieve redness and produce a soothing effect for a few hours, that is just about all that can be said for them. The fact is that normal eyes do not need cleansing, soothing, or refreshing by solutions of vasoactive and antiseptic chemicals. Simple irritation disappears of its own accord in about a day. No synthetic solution can match natural tears for washing away small bits of dust, dirt, or other irritating matter. And human tears contain an enzyme that has mild antibacterial properties at least as effective as those of the commercial eye solutions.

But essential uselessness is not the only criticism to be made of eyewashes. A more important fault is that their continued use may lead to the neglect of symptoms that indicate serious trouble. One of the most severe disorders that eye discomfort may signal is glaucoma. It is estimated that in the United States 2 million people over thirty-five have this disease, and about 14 percent of all blindness is caused by it.

Glaucoma is an eye disease (the cause of which remains unknown) manifested by an increase in pressure within the eyeball. The elevated pressure proceeds to affect the visual apparatus of the eye, creating characteristic blindspots and leading in some cases to blindness. In closed-angle (acute) glaucoma, the eye becomes red and extremely painful and requires emergency treatment by an ophthalmologist in a hospital setting.

Persons with narrow anterior chambers (which may or may not be detected in routine eye examination) are predisposed to acute glaucoma. Some medications—including OTC eye solutions containing a vasoconstrictor—may precipitate a first attack of closed-angle glaucoma in those who are unaware of their susceptibility to the disease. Other medications that may trigger an attack include antihistamines, which may be present in preparations used for the relief of colds and for motion sickness, and in OTC sleep remedies; certain drugs taken for gastrointestinal spasms; and tricyclic antidepressants. Because of its painful onset, such an attack is not likely to be neglected. But in simple (chronic) glaucoma the only complaint may be vague eye discomfort without redness or pain—precisely the kind of eye discomfort for which some people may use OTC remedies.

Many people have simple glaucoma without knowing it, and the disease can do irreparable damage to the sight without ever causing marked discomfort. Because of the prevalence of glaucoma in the adult population, the National Society for the Prevention of Blindness and practicing eye specialists as well urge glaucoma screening tests during periodic health checkups for adults over thirty-five (sooner for diabetics). If detected early, glaucoma can be treated—and sight saved. When you have your next eye checkup, it may be wise to ask the ophthalmologist or optometrist whether you are susceptible to closed-angle glaucoma and thus should be wary of using the above-mentioned drugs.

In the fall of 1978, the Food and Drug Administration approved a new drug for the treatment of glaucoma. Used as eyedrops, the drug timolol (Timoptic) is highly effective. Its long-lasting action means that patients need to use it only twice a day as opposed to four to six times a day for other topical medications for glaucoma.

Smarting, burning, itching, and inflammation of the whites of the eye (conjunctivitis) and eyelids (blepharitis) are often caused by infection with bacteria or viruses or by allergies to dust, pollens, or molds. Most bacterial infections of the eyes can be cured fairly quickly by antibiotic drops or ointments prescribed by a physician. Authorities believe that viral infections of the eyes occur more frequently than previously supposed. Conjunctivitis, often referred to as "pink eye," frequently occurs a few days after swimming in a pool, even an adequately chlorinated pool. The discomfort may be severe. The infection which can be highly contagious, usually requires a visit to a physician for proper diagnosis and treatment.

An acute inflammatory disorder of the eyes may be in reality a local manifestation of a general infection. Reddening of the eyes and sensitivity to light are common with measles. It is not unusual for mild inflammation of the eyes to accompany viral respiratory infections. Chronic inflammation of certain parts of the eye may signal the onset of a systemic disease, such as rheumatoid arthritis or sarcoidosis.

Eye fatigue may result from errors of refraction, such as astigmatism, farsightedness, or nearsightedness; it may be associated with general fatigue, such as that resulting from a sleepless night. Simple irritation may be caused by smog, strong light, sea bathing, or bathing in chlorinated water. There are various diseases, such as hyperthyroidism, diabetes, and myasthenia gravis, that affect the eye muscles and lids, giving rise to eye fatigue or double vision.

It should be apparent from this brief catalog of the possible causes of common eye complaints that OTC eyewashes cannot eliminate or treat such causes. If any of these symptoms persists more than a day or so, the eyes should be examined by a physician.

For "tired" but otherwise healthy eyes, Consumers Union's medical consultants believe that temporary relief may also be obtained with such time-honored remedies as one or two drops of cold tap water, placed in the lower lid with a clean eye dropper, or the application of iced wet compresses for about fifteen minutes.

According to CU's medical consultants, a boric acid solution should never be used as an eyewash because of possible toxicity. Furthermore, such solutions have not been shown to be more effective than plain water for the relief of eye discomfort.

Beyond any claimed therapeutic effect, some of the OTC eye solutions seem to offer a cosmetic benefit: "Get the red out," says one ad for a topical vasoconstrictor. CU's medical consultants advise against using such products on a long-term basis. Such misuse risks a rebound effect in which the condition returns with increasing severity.

7
Indigestion and antacids

Over the years, antacid products have been promoted for a host of common ills—from simple heartburn or mild indigestion to bloating, cramps, "gas pains," and "morning sickness." At least 575 different tablets, liquids, powders, lozenges, gums, and pills compete to soothe our stomach complaints. Yet fewer than a dozen brands account for most of the advertising—and sales— in this more than $200 million market.

How safe and effective are these widely promoted brands? And how valid are the advertising claims for them? Exact answers are elusive, because "indigestion" is a catchall label for a variety of symptoms, and tests comparing the touted remedies often lack scientific validity.

Indigestion can be a temporary symptom following an elaborate meal, or a recurrent symptom signaling a more serious problem, such as peptic ulcer. It may result directly from one of several diseases of the upper digestive tract, or it may be a sign of some other disorder, such as motion sickness or coronary disease. In fact, heart pain is one of the most important causes of indigestion-like symptoms in middle-aged men. Indigestion may also be a side effect of many prescription drugs, particularly antibiotics, as well as cortisone and some antiarthritis medicines. Such symptoms can usually be helped by taking the medication on a full stomach or with milk, although this procedure may lessen the effectiveness of certain antibiotics (such as tetracycline) by reducing the absorption into the bloodstream. (When in doubt, consult your pharmacist or physician.)

The occasional digestive upset that follows overindulgence, a rough day at the office, or a family squabble is usually no cause for alarm and may be treated with a variety of familiar remedies, including ordinary baking soda in water. But there are three situations that call for immediate medical attention: Any single episode of severe or persistent discomfort, especially if accompanied by sweating, weakness, or breathlessness; any single episode accompanied by vomiting of blood; and repeated episodes of indigestion—no matter how mild. "Repeated" may mean as infrequently as a few times a month for several months. In such instances, self-medication with an antacid can be dangerous, because it may mask a serious disorder and thus delay essential medical treatment.

Even for illnesses in which antacids are an accepted part of therapy—such as peptic ulcer—self-medication without medical supervision can be hazardous. Although a physician may prescribe an antacid for the temporary relief of ulcer pain, the ulcer may still become worse and the patient must be closely observed. If perforation should occur, leakage of gastric or intestinal contents could cause intense pain, infection, shock, and even death. In short, indiscriminate use of antacids can involve serious perils—a fact that is rarely, if ever, noted in the ads for these nonprescription items.

One of the oldest and most familiar antacids is sodium bicarbonate (baking soda). It is currently a major ingredient of *Alka-Seltzer*—one of the top sellers in the antacid field—and of *Bromo Seltzer* and lesser known brands including *Bell-Ans,*

Brioschi, Eno, and *Fizrin.* Sodium bicarbonate is a potent and fast-acting antacid, but one of the least desirable for regular or frequent use. If taken daily for more than a few weeks by people with diminished kidney function, a bicarbonate-containing antacid may disturb the body's acid-base balance and cause the body fluids to become more alkaline than normal. Prolonged use of such an alkalinizing agent may even lead to formation of calcium stones in the kidney and may also contribute to recurrent urinary tract infections.

What's more, the amounts of sodium in *Alka-Seltzer* and *Bromo Seltzer* (see table on pages 98–99) can be harmful to individuals with hypertension or congestive heart failure or to anyone else who must restrict sodium intake for whatever reason. For example, a heart patient allowed only 1,000 to 2,000 milligrams (mg) of sodium daily would risk upsetting that regimen with a single dose of *Alka-Seltzer* or *Bromo Seltzer.* In a customary two-tablet dose, *Alka-Seltzer* contains 1,042 mg of sodium. *Bromo Seltzer* has 758 mg per level capful. (The recommended dose of *Bromo Seltzer* is "one or two level capfuls.") In short, because of hazards associated with both sodium and bicarbonate, antacids containing sodium bicarbonate should be limited strictly to healthy individuals—and only for occasional use.

The Food and Drug Administration (FDA) advisory panel on antacids, which published its report in April 1973, judged unsuitable for people on low-salt diets any antacid containing more than 115 mg of sodium per maximum daily dose. Because many people have undetected heart or kidney disorders and the prevalence of these conditions increases with age, the panel recommended that no more than 2,300 mg of sodium per day in antacids be taken by *anyone* over sixty years of age. Current labels on *Alka-Seltzer* include: "60 years of age or older, maximum dosage four tablets daily" (2,084 mg); and *Bromo Seltzer* labels warn: "not more than three capfuls if over 60 in a 24-hour period" (2,274 mg). Thus for those sixty years of age or older, both products specify a maximum dosage that falls within the recommended limits for sodium.

A disadvantage of *Alka-Seltzer* for regular use as an antacid is its aspirin content. Aspirin in an antacid can be dangerous, especially if taken for symptoms that stem from ulcers or other serious stomach disorders. The FDA panel concluded that antacid/aspirin combinations "are irrational for antacid use alone and therefore should not be labeled or marketed for such use." The occasional use of an antacid/aspirin combination to relieve the discomfort of a combined headache and upset stomach seems reasonable. But *repeated* use for treatment of this double affliction, or for relief of either set of symptoms, is not recommended by Consumer Union's medical consultants.

Over the years, CU's medical consultants have frequently advised against the regular use of *Alka-Seltzer* as an antacid. In their judgment, its continued popularity is a clear defeat for public health education. However, the findings of the FDA panel appear to have influenced the advertising for *Alka-Seltzer*. The product is promoted for those suffering simultaneously from headache and stomach upset who may wish to avoid taking both ordinary aspirin and a simple antacid. This theme may make more medical sense but, CU believes, the advertising should also include information about the hazards of repeated use.

In 1974, Miles Laboratories, the makers of *Alka-Seltzer*, began nationwide distribution of *Alka-Seltzer Without Aspirin*. According to the manufacturer, the only changes in formulation were elimination of *Alka-Seltzer*'s aspirin content and inclusion of potassium bicarbonate. Miles also introduced a chewable product, *Alka-2*, containing calcium carbonate.

While *Bromo Seltzer* trails well behind *Alka-Seltzer* in advertising and sales, it runs neck and neck in dubious safety credentials. Like *Alka-Seltzer, Bromo Seltzer* adds an analgesic to a potent dose of antacid. Its analgesic—acetaminophen— does not irritate the stomach as much as aspirin does, but it is not necessary in an antacid. In 1977, as a result of FDA recommendations, *Bromo Seltzer* was reformulated and no longer contains phenacetin (which has been banned from OTC remedies—see page 19) or caffeine.

The judgment of CU's medical consultants is that ordinary sodium bicarbonate neutralizes stomach acid as adequately as any of the costlier products containing it. People who would rather take an effervescent product, however, should be careful to choose one that is basically a straight antacid. Such products as *Brioschi* and *Eno,* for example, contain no other active ingredients than antacids. Both are high in sodium bicarbonate, however, and consequently should *not* be used regularly or frequently by healthy people, and not at all by those on low-salt diets. *Fizrin,* which contains aspirin and sodium carbonate as well as sodium bicarbonate, is generally similar in composition to *Alka-Seltzer.* Goodman and Gilman's *The Pharmacological Basis of Therapeutics* reports that sodium carbonate "is obsolete as an antacid because it is highly alkaline and irritating, and can even be corrosive." Accordingly, CU's medical consultants judge *Fizrin* to be an even worse choice than *Alka-Seltzer* for regular use as an antacid.

Until a few years ago, calcium carbonate prescribed in powder form was the antacid of choice of many physicians; it provided rapid action and a high neutralizing capacity. Calcium carbonate is still the principal antacid in numerous over-the-counter products. However, this compound tends to cause constipation; and, more seriously, its prolonged and excessive use may raise calcium in the blood to undesirable levels and cause impaired kidney function and possible stone formation.

Ingredients of selected antacid products

Product	Form	Major antacid
Alka-Seltzer	tablet	sodium bicarbonate
Bromo Seltzer	granules	sodium bicarbonate
Di-Gel	liquid	aluminum hydroxide; magnesium carbonate
	tablet	aluminum hydroxide; magnesium carbonate
Gelusil	suspension or tablet	aluminum hydroxide; magnesium hydroxide
Maalox	suspension	aluminum hydroxide; magnesium hydroxide
Mylanta	suspension or tablet	aluminum hydroxide; magnesium hydroxide
Phillips' Milk of Magnesia	suspension or tablet	magnesium hydroxide
Rolaids	tablet	dihydroxyaluminum sodium carbonate
Tums	tablet	calcium carbonate

*Antacids with more than 115 mg of sodium per maximum daily dose should not be used by patients on low-salt diets, except with the advice and supervision of a physician. In general, products containing 9 mg or less of sodium per normal dose are preferred for low-salt diets.

Other antacid	Nonantacid	Approximate sodium content*
citric acid; potassium bicarbonate	aspirin	521 mg per tablet
citric acid	acetaminophen	758 mg per capful
magnesium hydroxide	simethicone	1.7 mg per teaspoon
magnesium hydroxide	simethicone	10.6 mg per tablet
—	simethicone	0.16 mg per teaspoon; 1.7 mg per tablet
—	**	0.5 mg per teaspoon†
—	simethicone	0.054 mg per teaspoon; 0.043 mg per tablet
—	—	(not specified)
—	—	53 mg per tablet
—	—	2.7 mg per tablet

**Maalox Plus* contains simethicone.
†*Maalox No. 1* contains 0.84 mg of sodium per tablet; *Maalox No. 2* contains 1.8 mg per tablet; *Maalox Plus* (suspension or tablet) contains 0.5 mg per teaspoon or 1.4 mg per tablet.

The likelihood of developing high blood calcium levels appears to increase for those who frequently consume large amounts of milk or who have kidney problems to begin with.

To prevent harmful effects, the FDA antacids panel advised against taking more than 8 grams (8,000 mg) of calcium carbonate daily. Labeling proposed by the panel, and subsequently enacted, limits this dosage level to a maximum period of two weeks, "except under the advice and supervision of a physician." Currently, each *Tums* tablet contains approximately 500 mg of calcium carbonate; thus the maximum daily dosage of *Tums,* for example, should not exceed sixteen tablets, nor should use at this level extend beyond two weeks. The experience of CU's medical consultants indicates that many current users exceed these amounts.

Research has suggested that calcium carbonate can cause an "acid rebound." A study published in *The New England Journal of Medicine* in September 1973 indicated that significant increases in stomach acid production followed the ingestion by healthy people of as little as 500 mg of calcium carbonate. (Some of the brands whose recommended single dosage contains approximately 500 mg or more of calcium carbonate include *Alkets, Camalox, Dicarbosil, Titralac* liquid, and *Tums.*) Although the mechanism of this stomach acid release is unknown, that same study showed mild elevations in blood levels of gastrin, a hormone known to facilitate secretion of acid by the stomach. Consequently, the effect of antacids containing calcium may be self-defeating. CU's medical consultants advise against the routine use of antacids containing calcium carbonate, particularly those with significant amounts in their formulation.

Tums and *Rolaids* are both available in convenient roll packs, but there the similarity ends. In contrast to *Tums,* whose main antacid ingredient is calcium carbonate, *Rolaids* contains an antacid that combines properties of sodium bicar-bonate and aluminum hydroxide. While *Tums* is low in sodium (2.7 mg), *Rolaids* contains 53 mg of it per tablet—which is high for anyone who must restrict salt intake. Occasional use of either *Tums* or *Rolaids* presents little hazard. However, because of the calcium content of *Tums* and the sodium bicar-bonate properties of *Rolaids,* neither product is suitable for frequent, long-term use.

Pepto-Bismol liquid and tablets are not antacids, but rather aids "for digestive upsets"—whatever that means. They contain bismuth subsalicylate as their main ingredi-ent. *The Pharmacological Basis of Therapeutics* observes: "While insoluble bismuth compounds are still employed for supposed effects in the gastrointestinal tract, there is no evi-dence of their efficacy." The FDA advisory panel on anta-cids has prohibited label claims such as "for heartburn and acid indigestion." In view of potential side effects, including possible darkening of the tongue and blackening of the stool (which may mask gastrointestinal bleeding from an ulcer), CU's medical consultants advise against the use of *Pepto-Bismol* products.

In contrast to its warnings on bicarbonate, calcium, and sodium, the FDA panel found two common antacid ingredi-ents to be relatively nonhazardous. It judged aluminum com-pounds to be safe in the amounts usually taken and placed no dosage restrictions on them. It reached a similar verdict on magnesium compounds, except for patients with chronic kid-ney disease. Since these patients have less ability to eliminate magnesium from their body, the panel set a dosage limit in such cases.

The best known aluminum compound is aluminum hydrox-ide. *Amphojel* is one of the few examples of an antacid using aluminum hydroxide as its single active ingredient. Although its onset of effect is slow and its neutralizing capacity variable, aluminum hydroxide provides relatively prolonged antacid action. Aluminum compounds also decrease the absorption of phosphate in the intestine, an effect that may benefit kidney patients who have elevated blood phosphate levels. However, aluminum compounds may cause severe constipation, which has tended to limit the popularity of products depending on this antacid ingredient alone. To offset the drawback, aluminum hydroxide is often combined with magnesium compounds, which tend to have a laxative effect. (For a discussion of magnesium/aluminum products, see below.)

Magnesium hydroxide may be purchased as milk of magnesia, a simple antacid available under this generic name at any pharmacy. The main ingredient in any brand of milk of magnesia, magnesium hydroxide, is an effective and generally safe antacid. The problem with such products, however, is their laxative effect. Ordinarily, the antacid dosage of, for example, *Phillips' Milk of Magnesia* is only one to three teaspoons (or two to four tablets). The same product is advertised as a laxative at a dosage of two to four tablespoons (or six to eight tablets). Consequently, people who repeat the antacid dosage or who are more susceptible than others to its laxative action may experience an unwanted side effect.

People with chronic kidney disorders should not use milk of magnesia or other magnesium antacids on a regular basis except under the supervision of a physician. More than three teaspoons (or more than four tablets) per day of *Phillips' Milk of Magnesia* exceeds the safe limit for magnesium set by the FDA panel for chronic kidney patients.

CU's medical consultants believe that the antacid products most likely to offer relative safety and a minimum of side effects—particularly for long-term use—are those containing aluminum hydroxide and magnesium hydroxide or trisilicate.

Products containing both aluminum hydroxide and magnesium hydroxide include *Aludrox, Creamalin, Kudrox, Maalox, Maxamag Suspension, Syntrogel,* and *WinGel.* Most of these brands are available either as a liquid or in tablet form. In addition to employing aluminum and magnesium hydroxides together, *Di-Gel* and *Mylanta* contain simethicone (an anti-flatulent, not an antacid), which the manufacturers say may help to relieve "gas pains."

Other products combine magnesium trisilicate with aluminum hydroxide. As in aluminum compounds, the antacid action of magnesium trisilicate is slow in onset but is of comparatively long duration. Brands with this combination include *A-M-T, Pama, Trimagel,* and *Trisogel.* (These products, too, can be obtained in either liquid or suspension formulation.)

A study in *The New England Journal of Medicine,* published in May 1973, reported that products with magnesium hydroxide are faster in onset of action and higher in acid-neutralizing capacity than those with magnesium trisilicate. Both compounds, however, were judged effective by the FDA panel. One product, *Magnatril,* apparently "just to be sure," combines aluminum hydroxide with *both* magnesium hydroxide and trisilicate.

Among the most important findings of the FDA panel were its conclusions about product claims. The panel declared that antacids can relieve heartburn, sour stomach, or acid indigestion but that any other claim is unfounded. Assertions that a product can alleviate nervous or emotional disturbances, "acidosis," "food intolerance," or morning sickness of pregnancy were found untruthful or inaccurate. Also judged unproven or unlikely were claims for relieving such symptoms as "gas," nausea, upset stomach, "full feeling," and the like. In short, the panel concluded that an antacid performs only one function: It neutralizes acid—period.

In addition to limiting label claims, the monograph on antacids prepared by the FDA (based on the panel report) lists the active ingredients the panel found to be safe and effective. For some of these ingredients the panel set the maximum amount to be allowed in an antacid product. The monograph, published in final form in June 1974, has the force of law.

Decisions by the panel about effective ingredients, dosage levels, product claims, and labeling should help you make a more rational selection of an antacid preparation. CU's medical consultants urge you to consider the following guidelines when you think you need an antacid.

- Do not use any antacid regularly for more than a few weeks, except with the advice and supervision of a physician.
- Restrict sodium bicarbonate or calcium carbonate antacids to occasional use only, and give preference to products with aluminum and magnesium ingredients.
- If you are on a sodium-restricted diet, stick to an antacid low in sodium. Check the table on pages 98–99; if necessary, ask your pharmacist or physician for a recommendation.
- The liquid and suspension forms of an antacid seem to be more effective than the equivalent dose in tablets. To be effective, tablets must be thoroughly sucked or chewed; otherwise they may not dissolve completely in the stomach before entering the small intestine.
- If a certain food or beverage consistently causes stomach upsets, it makes more sense to cut out the troublemaker than to resort to medicine to relieve the symptoms. Should you fail to identify the culprit in your diet that is the probable cause of abdominal discomfort, or should you be uncertain, it may be wise to seek medical advice.
- And most important, if repeated or painful episodes of indigestion occur, stop self-diagnosis and self-medication and consult your physician.

▪ A special word for women who are pregnant: Because pregnant women must be careful to restrict aspirin intake during the last three months of pregnancy (see page 31), they should shun antacid preparations containing aspirin. They also should be cautious about frequent use of antacids with a high sodium content. Even though it now has been shown that sodium is not generally harmful to pregnant women and, in fact, does not increase the hazard of toxemia, the ingestion of excessive amounts of sodium is a practice that would be sanctioned by few, if any, obstetricians. CU's medical consultants urge pregnant women to check with their doctors before taking any antacid preparation to relieve symptoms of stomach distress—and for that matter before taking *any* drug (see Chapter 22).

8
Constipation and diarrhea

Most cases of constipation cure themselves without the use of drugs, although there are circumstances in which a mild laxative can be beneficial and relatively harmless. When, for example, there is temporary difficulty in evacuation due to emotional stress, traveling, or change in diet, there is no harm in taking a mild laxative for a day or two. And in some cases of chronic constipation—if it definitely has been proved to exist and there is no organic cause—a physician may suggest a laxative to help relieve the condition. But the widespread overdependence on laxatives, which supports the sale of more than 700 different over-the-counter (OTC) laxative products, can be explained only by an equally widespread misunderstanding of constipation and the drugs used to treat it.

There is no such thing as a perfect, natural, or entirely harmless laxative. All types have some disadvantages. Moreover, the distinction that the advertisers of commercial products make between mild laxatives and harsh cathartics is highly deceptive. *Any* material taken by mouth to promote evacuation of the intestine is a cathartic drug; a laxative is simply a mild cathartic. But one person's laxative may be another's cathartic. And in the same person a drug can act as a laxative at one time and act more like a cathartic at another.

There can be no doubt that laxatives have contributed more to the ills and discomforts of mankind than the condition they are supposed to relieve. Instances of a ruptured appendix with peritonitis have been recorded in patients who assumed their abdominal pain was caused by constipation and so dosed themselves with laxatives. Constipation is rarely associated with severe abdominal pain. Nor does the presence of pain mean the bowels need to be cleaned out.

Who has not heard that, at the beginning of a cold or an attack of grippe, flu, or acute tonsillitis, a cathartic should be taken? This myth is a holdover from the Middle Ages when "a dose of the salts" was supposed to cure everything from ague to plague. Yet catharsis does not prevent, cure, or lessen the severity of these illnesses or any other acute illness. In acute illnesses, constipation may simply be associated with dehydration, poor intake of food, or prolonged inactivity. To purge a patient who is already suffering from depleted fluid reserves is foolish—and may even be disastrous.

No organ of the body is as misunderstood, maltreated, and fussed over as the digestive tract. It has been purged, irrigated, lavaged, massaged, and pummeled, all in the name of that great American obsession, the daily bowel movement. It is commonly believed that the waste matter left after digestion has been completed must be expelled twenty-four to forty-eight hours after the food is eaten. The fallacy of this impression was revealed in an experiment supervised by the late Walter C. Alvarez, M.D. A group of healthy young medical students swallowed sets of gelatin capsules containing many small glass beads. The results were interesting. Two of the students passed about 85 percent of the beads in twenty-four hours; most took four days to eliminate three-fourths of the beads; some passed only half of the beads in nine days.

Alvarez further observed that those who passed the majority of the beads in twenty-four hours had poorly formed stools containing undigested material. Those with a slower rate usually had well-formed stools showing evidence of good digestion. Some of the participants with the slower rates had believed that they were constipated.

Alvarez has likened the colon and its fecal contents to a railroad siding on which three freight cars are standing. Every day a new car arrives and bumps the end one off, leaving three again. But occasionally one arrives at the siding with such force that it bumps all three off, and then three days must elapse before the siding is full again. In other words, when the colon is cleaned out by a purge or large bowel movement, nothing more should be expected for several days.

Nor does everyone operate on a once-a-day schedule. It is common to find people in perfect health who defecate two or three times a day, and others who have a single evacuation every two or three days without the slightest ill effect. There are many individuals who have bowel movements at still longer intervals without any impairment of health.

Constipation, then, cannot be defined in terms of a daily bowel movement, but must be related to each person's normal functioning. Missing a few bowel movements should cause no panic. After a few days, things generally return to normal, and the rhythm is reestablished.

When true chronic constipation is present, it may result from overemphasis on toilet training in childhood, improper bowel habits, crowded living conditions, poor diet, or the like. A small percentage of patients with constipation have an organic disease such as diverticulitis or cancer. This cause is most likely to be found in adults who previously have had regular and satisfactory evacuation but then begin to experience a persistent change in the character or frequency of bowel movements.

To investigate the possibility of organic disease, a physician may directly observe the rectum and lower bowel through a lighted tube called a sigmoidoscope. The physician also may have a radiologist perform a barium-enema X-ray examination to inspect the remainder of the large bowel. But to repeat, constipation caused by an organic disease is not common. In general, if constipation has been present for a number of years, the likelihood is that the condition is not due to serious disease.

More often, bowel dysfunction reflects emotional stresses. Such influences on the colon may be important, and also quite perverse. In one person they may speed up bowel transit time for ingested foodstuffs and cause diarrhea with occasional mucus in the stool. In another they may slow bowel activity and cause hard, dry, and infrequent stools. In a third they may lead to intestinal spasms perceived as painful abdominal cramps, with alternating periods of diarrhea and constipation.

When these conditions persist or recur, they are known collectively as the irritable colon syndrome. This is the likely diagnosis in the case of long-standing bowel complaints associated with worry, fear, and anxiety. The irritable colon syndrome is an emotionally triggered disorder in which the intestine functions like a barometer. Irregular peristalsis results not only in abdominal pains and distention but also in excessive passage of gas; and hard stools often alternate with looser stools. Treatment of the irritable colon syndrome calls for treatment of the underlying psychological disorder and whatever else serves to cushion the individual's anxiety. (Bloody stools, which are not usually associated with the irritable colon syndrome, always require consultation with a physician.)

The irritable colon syndrome is no longer considered the only cause for complaints of bloating, gaseous distention, and intermittent loose stools. It has been shown that for some people a more likely explanation may be what formerly was called an intestinal "allergy." A physician may discover through careful questioning that the discomfort is due to a food intolerance. A frequent cause is the lack of an intestinal enzyme—lactase—which is essential for the proper digestion of milk products. These foods tend to precipitate episodes of abdominal discomfort. The ingestion of certain other foods can cause similar patterns such as the florid diarrhea, experienced by patients with nontropical sprue and celiac disease—an intestinal malfunction caused by intolerance to gluten (the insoluble protein constituent of wheat and other grains).

Unfortunately, the symptoms of an irritable colon are not always evident. For example, the emotional factors responsible for bowel dysfunction may not be obvious, so that it is not always possible for the sufferers to know that their constipation or diarrhea is of this type. This is another reason why proper diagnosis is important before a course of treatment for chronic constipation or diarrhea is begun.

Some medications frequently cause loose, watery bowel movements. The most common offenders include such antibiotics as lincomycin, ampicillin, and tetracycline. Also capable of provoking diarrhea are some magnesium-containing antacids (see page 102) and ascorbic acid (vitamin C).

If an attack of diarrhea does not subside in a day, or if diarrhea is accompanied at any time by fever, severe abdominal pain, or bloody stools, self-medication is not advisable, and the patient should consult a physician. In any case, a person suffering from diarrhea should drink plenty of liquids to offset loss of fluids in the watery stools. Decreasing the amount of roughage (or bulk producers) in the diet—for example, cutting out most raw fruits and raw vegetables—plus the time-honored reliance on rice and bananas may reduce the severity of the attack.

OTC preparations commonly used for acute diarrhea, such

as kaolin/pectin mixtures (*Kaopectate* and *Pektamalt,* among others), are less effective than antidiarrheal drugs containing codeine or opium. The latter are narcotic drugs, which require a prescription. Physicians may prescribe a small quantity of codeine tablets, tincture of opium, powdered opium in capsules, paregoric, diphenoxylate (Lomotil), or loperamide (Imodium). These drugs, which are all narcotics or closely related synthetic derivatives, are effective in relieving diarrhea reasonably promptly. In the amounts used for occasional diarrheal attacks, they should present no problem of dependency. Consumers Union's medical consultants warn against the use of diphenoxylate and loperamide for infants and young children. Toxicity has been observed with minimal dosage. Their safety for use by pregnant women has not been established. They should be used with caution, if at all, in acute infectious diarrhea.

The affliction commonly referred to as "acute gastroenteritis" usually involves two or three days of diarrhea, along with fever and general malaise. It is thought to be viral in origin. Healthy individuals are able to withstand such illness with only minor discomfort. The very young and the very old, regardless of their health, tend to fare less well. Because they need adequate fluid replacement, some may even require hospitalization.

Most attacks of diarrhea tend to be self-limited, with the symptoms relieved (with or without medication) in a few days. However, diarrhea can be protracted, lasting more than a week. In the beginning stages underlying causes of protracted diarrhea, such as amebic dysentery or ulcerative colitis, may be difficult to diagnose. Because specific therapy for such diseases must often await diagnosis, it is important, when diarrhea is prolonged, to have microscopic and bacteriological examinations made of the stool, as well as sigmoidoscopic examination of the rectum. X rays of the bowel also may be necessary.

The cause of chronic constipation is frequently more prosaic. Something as simple as improper toilet habits may be an underlying cause. When the urge to defecate is disregarded, the sensation passes. It usually returns again during the day, especially after meals, but if the call is consistently disobeyed day after day, the rectum may eventually fail to signal the need for evacuation. The result may be severe constipation.

Why is the call disregarded? It may be suppressed, or it may be overwhelmed by other and stronger stimuli, similar to loss of one's appetite on hearing a piece of bad news. It also may be neglected because of the pressure of school or work, or perhaps because there is a morning train to catch, or only one bathroom for a large family.

The misuse of laxatives is another important cause of chronic constipation. Whatever the original reason for starting it, repeated purgation in time brings changes in the lining and muscle tone of the bowel; the lining can become irritated and inflamed, and with long-continued catharsis muscular reflexes can become so diminished that stronger and stronger stimulation is required to produce activity. Moreover, there are comparatively few users of cathartics who have not suffered from fissure of the anus or hemorrhoids (see Chapter 9). Such ailments often make defecation so painful that the sufferer tends to postpone a visit to the toilet, with the same results as those occurring in a person who is too busy. Chronic laxative users may also unknowingly be depleting their body of potassium, resulting in muscle weakness.

Of major importance as a possible cause of constipation are many OTC and prescription drugs in common use today. Antacids may often be a source of difficulty (see Chapter 7). Among the prescription drugs the most notorious offenders are narcotics such as codeine, opium, and oxycodone (the active ingredient in Percodan). Another class of compounds capable of causing constipation includes those affecting the parasympathetic nervous system. Among these drugs are gastrointestinal antispasmodics such as propantheline (Pro-Banthine), antidepressants such as imipramine (Tofranil), and major tranquilizers such as chlorpromazine (Thorazine). Should constipation become severe after the use of these drugs, a physician may decrease dosage or switch to another medication in order to relieve that distressing side effect.

Against this background of the cause—more properly, causes—of constipation, some rational approaches to treatment suggest themselves. If you think you have chronic constipation, the first thing to do is to stop taking laxatives. Many people who have done so at the insistence of a doctor have been surprised to find that, after a few days or a week, the bowels begin to move effectively again. For temporary constipation, the obvious thing to do is nothing; let nature take its course, and the condition will cure itself. But some people complain of headache or sluggishness or they just plain worry if they don't have a regular bowel movement; for such people it may be less harmful to use a laxative once in a while than to fret. The mildest laxative that produces results is the best choice (see page 116).

Some people may find it more natural, if not as convenient, to use an enema instead of a laxative. As authorities have been saying for many years, it does seem unreasonable to upset 25 feet of intestine with a cathartic when the trouble is in the last 8 inches—the rectum and anal canal. An enema consisting of a pint of tepid tap water is generally sufficient. While relatively expensive, prepackaged disposable enemas (e.g., *Fleet*) can be a convenience. But too frequent use of enemas—even once a week, for some people—can result in an inability to initiate a bowel movement without recourse to an enema. (High colonic enemas, incidentally, are an antiquated, useless, and sometimes harmful procedure. They do not cure habitual constipation or remove "toxins," and do not in any way promote health or prolong life.)

Glycerin suppositories have also been employed to stimulate evacuation of the rectum without disturbing the rest of the bowel. Their occasional use does no harm, but most physicians believe that for many individuals frequent use of suppositories can cause irritation both of the anus and of the mucous membrane of the rectum.

Some people might find it helpful to add roughage (or bulk producers) to their diet in the form of fruits, vegetables, and whole-grain cereals. Remember, however, that the human intestinal tract is not constructed like that of a plant-eating animal. It is able to digest a wide variety of foods, but not the diet of a cow or rabbit. Also, there are individual idiosyncrasies. Some people can eat a high percentage of roughage without the slightest inconvenience. The same meal can produce distress in others. If pain, distention, mucus in the stool, or other evidence of irritation occurs, a physician should be consulted.

Among the more valuable foods for roughage are bran, spinach, raw carrots, and whole fruit. Bran, often promoted for the relief of constipation, may be useful particularly to those who do not object to immediate and dramatic results. Cereals with the highest bran content include Kellogg's *All-Bran* and *Bran Buds* and Post's and Kellogg's *40% Bran Flakes* and *Raisin Bran.* Prunes, the traditional friend of the constipated, provide bulk and stimulate peristalsis. Peristalsis may also be aided through use of prune extract or prune juice.

The role of exercise in the treatment of constipation has been exaggerated, but it may divert one's thoughts from working cares or household worries, thus conferring the sense of relaxation that facilitates a bowel movement. Massaging the abdominal muscles is a waste of time as therapy for constipation. And there is little value in drinking large quantities of water—even hot water flavored with lemon. However, any of these measures may have an important psychological effect.

If simple measures don't clear up constipation within a week or so, the trouble very likely is true chronic constipation, and a doctor's help is needed. Rational treatment must be based on the cause, and that can be established for sure only through a physical examination and careful questioning. A doctor takes daily living habits and diet into account. Often a laxative is prescribed, as a temporary measure, to promote evacuation while the patient tries to reestablish a normal bowel routine. The laxative may then be gradually withdrawn.

In 1975 a Food and Drug Administration (FDA) advisory panel reviewed OTC laxatives. According to the panel's report, 25 percent of the eighty-one laxative ingredients submitted for review were judged unsafe or ineffective, and 20 percent needed further study.

Most of the ingredients judged unsafe or ineffective are no longer included in many of the products currently on the market. And some of the products that do contain them are being reformulated as a result of the panel's report. (*Carter's Little Pills,* for example, has been reformulated without podophyllum, an ingredient the panel found to be unsafe.)

Ingredients judged by the panel to lack "medical or scientific rationale" included capsicum (as in *Veracolate* and *Caroid and Bile Salts*), ginger (as in *Merit Cathartics*), and vitamins and minerals (as in *Geriplex FS* and *Imibicoll with Vitamin B1*). The panel recommended that labels list not only the quantity of each active ingredient in a recommended dose but also all inactive ingredients as well. It recommended that ingredients judged unsafe or ineffective or lacking in medical or scientific rationale be eliminated from OTC laxative products.

CU's medical consultants suggest that you avoid laxatives containing ingredients that act as bowel stimulants, unless advised by a physician. These drugs include phenolphthalein *(Ex-Lax, Feen-A-Mint),* senna *(Fletcher's Castoria, Senokot),* bisacodyl *(Dulcolax),* and cascara *(Cas-Evac).* All these agents stimulate peristalsis and are capable of producing severe painful cramping. The FDA panel has recommended that stimulant laxatives be labeled with this warning: "Prolonged or continued use of this product can lead to laxative dependency and loss of normal bowel function. Serious side effects from prolonged use or overuse may occur."

Another class of laxatives, which also produces its effects by increasing peristalsis, includes saline (salt) cathartics. The most popular salts used are magnesium citrate (citrate of magnesia), magnesium hydroxide (milk of magnesia), and sodium phosphate *(Buffered Laxative, Fleet, Sal Hepatica).* Results with these laxatives can be dramatic, depending on the dose used. Patients with chronic kidney disease, who may have difficulty in excreting magnesium, should be wary about using milk of magnesia. And patients on salt-restricted diets should avoid laxatives containing sodium.

CU's medical consultants recommend that—if you must resort to a laxative—you restrict yourself to a bulk-producing laxative or a stool softener. According to the FDA panel report, "Bulk-forming laxatives are among the safest of laxatives." (Most of them should be taken with a full glass of water to guard against the remote possibility of intestinal obstruction.) Bulk-producing laxatives, such as pysillium preparations *(Effersyllium Instant Mix, Konsyl, L.A. Formula, Metamucil Powder, Metamucil Instant Mix, Mucilose Flakes,* and *Mucilose Granules),* tend to cause fewer unpleasant side effects than bowel irritants. Note, however, that *L.A. Formula, Metamucil Powder,* and *Mucilose Granules* each has an equal amount of sugar plus the active ingredient. And salt-restricted dieters should note the fact that *Metamucil Instant Mix* contains a considerable quantity of sodium.

Semisynthetic cellulose derivatives are being used increasingly as bulk-forming laxatives. They include, for example, *Cellothyl* and *Hydrolose*. The correct dosage for cellulose derivatives, according to the panel, is four to six grams daily, taken with a full glass of water. *Cellothyl* requires at least eight tablets a day to reach the panel's recommended dosage; package directions recommend between three and nine tablets a day. *Hydrolose* should be taken as directed for proper dosage. These products are also available by generic name rather than brand name.

Stool softeners work for some people, but not for all. These detergent products act to permit fluids to penetrate the stool, and increase its water content. Dioctyl sodium (or calcium) sulfosuccinate is the main detergent or softener in clinical use, and is marketed under such brand names as *Colace, Coloctyl, Dio Medicone, Disonate, Doxinate,* and *Surfak.*

Mineral oil (an emollient) has had many loyal fans, particularly among older people. However, use of mineral oil over time —especially by the elderly or disabled—may lead to lipid pneumonia, a chronic condition caused by inhalation of oil into the lungs. Because of this and other disadvantages such as rectal leakage and interference with the body's absorption of vitamins A, D, E, and K, mineral oil is no longer a laxative of choice. The drawbacks of mineral oil, however, can be minimized by taking the smallest effective dose (about one tablespoon for an adult) on an empty stomach and by not lying down for at least half an hour after ingestion. Because the absorption of mineral oil can be facilitated by dioctyl sodium sulfosuccinate, these two agents should not be used at the same time.

The brand names on the preceding pages by no means

exhaust the list of laxatives marketed through drugstores and supermarkets. In addition to the single-ingredient preparations identified above, there is a large contingent of combination-type laxatives. Shoppers may find products combining a stool softener with a bulk laxative, or a bowel irritant with an emollient. As always, consumers are urged to read the label carefully. CU's medical consultants advise buying a product with only one active ingredient. Although the FDA panel would allow some products with two active laxative ingredients (but no more than two) to remain on the market, the panel agrees that a single-ingredient product is safest.

The laxative market is swamped with label claims that, in the panel's opinion, should be changed. A laxative label should not make assertions about general benefits for good health, regularity or the relief of "indigestion," "headaches," or "excessive belching." Instead, it should identify the product as a laxative for the "short-term relief of constipation." Nor should the label warn against the hazards of constipation, because such warnings are "unproven and thus unacceptable," according to the panel. Also forbidden would be any suggestion that taking a laxative is somehow natural. The panel points out that taking a laxative is never natural. And the label should not suggest that the laxative is particularly appropriate for individuals of a certain sex or age. If that last recommendation is accepted, *Correctol* could no longer print on its label, "The Woman's Gentle Laxative," nor could *Fletcher's Castoria* claim to be "for children."

Yogurt and acidophilus milk once had quite a vogue for the treatment of bowel disorders, including constipation. The nutritive value of yogurt and other fermented milks is essentially the same as that of the whole milk from which they are made, hence they are good foods. But, although fermented milks have occasionally been reported to be successful in the treatment of mild constipation, they usually are not of much value. Nor is there any evidence to support the routine use of vitamin B_1, vitamin B_6, or any other vitamin in the treatment of habitual constipation.

Constipation in children requires special consideration. In the great majority of cases it is due to oversolicitous attitudes on the part of parents. When a child senses anxiety in a parent about bowel function, the child too may become tense and unable to relax, and relaxation is essential to a normal bowel movement.

If constipation develops in a child, what should be done? A good rule to follow in treating a child's constipation is "Don't." A child will not become ill from a temporary lapse, and in a day or two normal bowel activity usually reestablishes itself spontaneously. If constipation is due to an acute ailment, medical supervision and nursing care for the acute illness, not laxatives, are required. If constipation tends to recur, it may be due to improper diet or bowel habits, and a physician should be consulted. The prohibition of laxatives, suppositories, and enemas for most children with constipation cannot be too strongly urged.

Pregnant women are especially susceptible to constipation because of the direct pressure of the enlarged uterus on the rectum as well as the relaxing effect of elevated hormone levels on the muscles of the bowel. But a pregnant woman should not take laxatives or any medication routinely without consulting a physician. There's no harm, however, in adding some roughage to the diet.

2

Hemorrhoids and other anal disorders

Few areas of the body are associated with so many inhibitions, fears, and fixations as the rectum and the anus. The anus is the body opening through which solid waste matter (feces) passes from the rectum. It is composed of circular muscle fibers, and its many nerve endings render it a very sensitive area. The rectum is the portion of the lower bowel, just above the anus, which leads from that part of the large bowel known as the sigmoid colon. The anorectal area is susceptible to three major disorders—itching, bleeding, and pain—which, either singly or in combination, may eventually require medical evaluation.

Many people are reluctant to consult a physician about problems in the anorectal area—some because of shyness, others because of the fear that cancer might be to blame. In fact, cancer and other tumors practically never occur in the anus. They do develop in the rectum, often without causing pain or bleeding in the early stages. Prior to causing symptoms, tumors can be detected only through periodic, routine rectal examination by a physician, either digitally, or, preferably, with a lighted tube called a sigmoidoscope.

Most disorders in the anorectal region are nonmalignant and, if given timely medical care, can be relieved or cured quickly. The most common of these disorders is hemorrhoids.

Hemorrhoids, also called piles, are clusters of dilated, or varicose, veins in the lower rectum and anus. They usually occur after the age of thirty; it is likely that one-third or more of the population suffers from them. Many people have both internal hemorrhoids, which may bleed but are usually painless, and the external type, which can be very painful indeed.

When the blood flow slows in one of these distended veins, clotting occurs resulting in a painful condition known as a thrombosed hemorrhoid. The pain of a thrombosed hemorrhoid can be formidable, and is aggravated by sitting, walking, sneezing, or coughing. Relief from this acute condition usually takes place when the clot is released by means of spontaneous rupture of the vein or by a surgical incision. Warm sitz baths (see below) may also prove helpful, but they usually take at least several days to bring relief.

Perhaps the most important factor in the development of hemorrhoids is chronic constipation. Habitual forceful straining to move the bowels leads to congestion and stretching of the veins of the rectum and anus. Too frequent use of laxatives may cause explosive types of bowel movements, which over a period of time can produce the same undesirable results.

In women, hemorrhoids frequently occur during or after pregnancy, as a result of increased pressure in the anal and rectal veins. Many people have noticed that stools tend to be looser and more frequent after drinking alcohol and that such a change in bowel habits, even though temporary, may provoke an attack of piles. And people with occupations requiring constant sitting or standing, or lifting of heavy objects, may be prone to hemorrhoids. In others, thrombosed piles often show up right after exercise requiring unusual strain. Often no precipitating factor can be identified.

The pain of external hemorrhoids may be relieved considerably by warm sitz baths, three or four times daily, for fifteen minutes at a time. Sitting in a warm bath eases pain by relaxing the spasm of the sphincter muscles around the anus. Lying down also helps by eliminating the pressure caused by gravity. After bowel movements, gentle cleaning with tepid water is less irritating than using dry toilet paper.

Suppositories, although widely advertised, are of little proven value for either internal or external hemorrhoids. The most popular ingredients of such suppositories are bismuth salts, topical anesthetics such as benzocaine, vasoconstrictors such as ephedrine, and antiseptics such as benzethonium chloride. Although the vasoconstrictor drugs in a suppository may be capable of checking minor capillary bleeding, they cannot be relied upon to check bleeding from a varicose vein. The latter type of bleeding usually stops by itself in a day or two, as soon as the pressure within the vein is relieved. However, *all* cases of rectal bleeding—new, persistent, or recurrent— merit consultation with a physician.

Nor do suppositories have any beneficial effect on the pain of hemorrhoids. When a suppository is inserted in the anus, it passes by the painful hemorrhoids and slips upward beyond the pain-sensitive lower rectum before melting. If one must use a suppository, it might make more sense to make it into a paste and apply it directly to the anal area. Indeed, such over-the-counter ointments or salves may be useful medications when applied directly to painful or bleeding sites.

Ointments containing such anesthetic drugs as benzocaine, dibucaine, or tetracaine seem to have a mild pain- or itch-relieving effect in some cases of external hemorrhoids. There is no convincing evidence that the highly advertised *Preparation H*—an ointment reported to contain a material derived from yeast cells, shark liver oil, and phenylmercuric nitrate— is any more effective in relieving pain than other ointments.

According to *The Medical Letter,* "There is no acceptable evidence substantiating advertised claims that *Preparation H* can shrink hemorrhoids, reduce inflammation, and heal injured tissue."

External hemorrhoids will generally become symptom-free by themselves if bowel function is improved. Neither electrocoagulation nor chemical cauterization is considered good practice in treating hemorrhoids, because these methods do not cure and they may cause secondary hemorrhage. Injection treatment is no longer widely used.

Severe cases of bleeding or painful hemorrhoids may require surgery. In most instances, surgery cures existing hemorrhoids permanently. But, because not all the rectal or anal veins can be removed, there is always a possibility that new hemorrhoids will develop.

There are several new techniques for dealing with certain types of hemorrhoids, but not all medical authorities agree as to their effectiveness. These include anal dilatation treatments and cryotherapy (a method that involves quick freezing of the hemorrhoids with specially designed instruments). Wide publicity has been given to these procedures, and each has its ardent supporters. However, CU's medical consultants believe that more experience is required with these treatments before either can be accepted for routine medical use. Rubber-band application has gained acceptance as an office procedure for the treatment of certain types of hemorrhoids.

Hemorrhoids are not the only cause of anal itching. Occasionally, a definable and possibly treatable skin disorder in or around the anal canal is responsible. In other cases, itching may be a symptom of a disease, such as diabetes, or it may come from infestation of the intestines by pinworms or roundworms; these causes of itching are treatable. Many times, however, no specific cause can be established; psychological factors probably play a significant role in many cases of chronic anal itch.

A lack of knowledge of the specific cause of anal itching in most patients has led to the use of many treatments of doubtful value, including anesthetic ointments, alcohol injections, tattooing of the skin with mercury, X ray, and even more radical procedures, such as excision of the skin. But all these measures have been largely supplanted by the application of ointments and salves containing cortisone or one of its numerous derivatives. Although in most cases those who need to use the medication remain virtually free of symptoms, use must be continued for an indefinite period to achieve this effect.

This method generally is not effective in treating the anal itching caused by oral antibiotics—particularly such broad-spectrum antibiotics as tetracycline or ampicillin. Such an itch may develop not only during the course of antibiotic treatment, but as late as a week or two afterward. This type of anal itch may be very resistant to treatment of any kind, but it usually disappears spontaneously, although it may take a long time. The use of lactobacillus tablets or yogurt—although frequently resorted to—has been shown to be ineffective in both prevention and treatment of antibiotic-induced anal itch. Some physicians may administer an antifungal agent with the antibiotic, but convincing proof that this is effective is lacking.

Anal fissures, which are small tears in the skin surrounding the anus, can be a cause of rectal pain, itching, and bleeding. These fissures are usually small and inconspicuous, so diagnosis must almost always be made by a physician. Treatment of anal fissures generally consists in keeping the area clean by means of sitz baths. In the intervals between baths ordinary talcum powder must be used to keep the area dry. Cauterization by a physician may be necessary in persistent cases.

Not only may self-treatment of any of the various rectal and anal disorders with nonprescription ointments or suppositories aggravate the trouble and sensitize the skin, but as a result serious conditions may be overlooked. Persistent or recurring itching, pain, or bleeding in the anorectal area are symptoms that should not be ignored or treated in a casual fashion with OTC remedies. Each of these symptoms should be evaluated by a physician and treated appropriately.

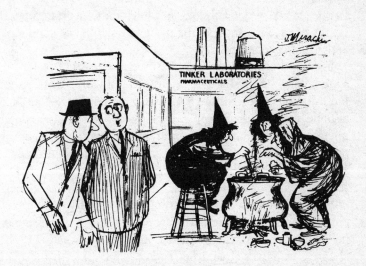

"We figure they may hit on something."

10
Acne

Although acne is not a fatal disease and only occasionally results in disfiguring scars, it can be a severe test of the emotional stamina of adolescents and their families. It usually comes at a time in life when increasing maturity is striving for expression, and appearance has assumed enormous importance. In our society—especially among adolescents—a clean, smooth skin, free of blemishes, seems to be the symbol of good looks and social acceptance.

For hundreds of years there has been a persistent belief that acne is in some mysterious way associated with sexual wishes, fantasies, or masturbation. This is simply not true. Acne may also be considered by some persons to be the stigmata of physical, mental, and social inferiority. This too is obviously false. Nevertheless, acne often causes immeasurable mental anguish to those afflicted. Advertisers of skin preparations for teenagers play on these anxieties in promoting their products.

Parents can make a real contribution if they try to help their children understand the nature of acne and not dismiss genuine concern as mere vanity. Armed with the information in this chapter, teenagers should be far less susceptible to the blandishments of misleading advertising.

Some self-help measures can play a role in acne care. But to understand why over-the-counter (OTC) medication is so problematical, one needs to know what factors lead to acne. *Acne* (eruption of the face) *vulgaris* (common) is primarily a disorder of the pilosebaceous units of certain areas of the skin. Each unit consists of a hair follicle—from which a hair shaft protrudes—and a sebaceous gland that secretes sebum (a whitish fatty substance) into the follicle and through the pores to the surface of the skin adjacent to the hair shaft. The normal follicle is lined with cells that age, die, and are easily extruded through the pores of the skin. In time, these cells are replaced by new cells and the cycle is repeated. Acne is caused by an abnormality in this orderly process of cell extrusion and replacement. When the skin pore in time becomes blocked with cellular debris, sebum, which is constantly being formed, cannot escape through the blocked pore onto the skin surface.

Corynebacterium acnes is the type of bacteria normally found within the follicle. Many dermatologists now believe that, as the amount of sebum within the pilosebaceous unit increases, these organisms release an enzyme that splits the sebum into smaller molecules called fatty acids. Disruption of the follicular wall then results from the direct irritant action of those fatty acids.

The primary lesions of acne are comedones (whiteheads): Collections of dead cells, sebum, and bacteria that clog the shaft of the hair follicle. On exposure to air, comedones darken (blackheads).

When disruption of the follicular wall occurs, additional lesions called papules and pustules appear. Papules are red, solid areas that protrude above the skin surface. Pustules are papules that extend deeper into the skin and contain pus. Pimple (or zit) is the usual lay term for papule or pustule.

There are large variations in the amount of sebum secreted

in different areas of the skin. The most active sebaceous glands are located in the scalp, followed in descending order of activity by the forehead, face, chest, and upper back. Except for the scalp, areas with the highest sebum production are the most frequent sites of acne.

As part of the normal maturing process, the sebaceous glands at puberty increase in size and secrete more sebum under the influence of increasing amounts of sex hormones, principally the male hormone testosterone, present in both males and females. The increase in sebum production, combined with obstruction of the pores, sets the stage for the development of acne. If the overactivity of the sebaceous glands or the plugging of the pores could be better controlled, acne might pose less of a problem.

Animal experiments have shown that the female sex hormones—progesterone and estrogen—as well as testosterone affect sebaceous activity. Testosterone and progesterone stimulate the sebaceous glands, while estrogen tends to reduce their activity. Estrogen, however, must be taken in fairly large doses —so large, in fact, as to produce undesirable side effects in the male—if it is to reduce sebaceous gland secretion to a degree that may be significant in acne. Consequently, the use of estrogen has been—and should be—reserved for females with severe potentially disfiguring acne. Such therapy, however, may be inadvisable in a still-growing female because it may stunt growth. When estrogen is prescribed for acne in a female who has attained full growth, it is often given in combination with a progestin (as in an oral contraceptive) in order to prevent irregular menstrual bleeding.

Unless acne is severe, however, a visit to the doctor is not usually necessary. Only one acne case in ten requires medical attention. Most mild or moderate cases respond to effective OTC medication (see pages 130–131) and to home care.

A wide variety of OTC acne products is available. Besides the creams, cleansers, lotions, soaps, powders, and gels one might expect, drugstores sell cleansing sticks, a variety of scrubs, impregnated towelettes, tablets, and many other items. Except for cosmetic agents designed solely to hide the lesions and to blend with the surrounding skin, many of these products contain the same time-honored medicaments tried by physicians over the years in managing this stubborn ailment.

Ingredients commonly used in OTC acne remedies and believed by most dermatologists to be of some value are benzoyl peroxide, salicylic acid, sulfur, and resorcinol. Of these, benzoyl peroxide is the most effective. It occurs in adequate concentrations in several OTC products (such as *Benoxyl, Loroxide, Oxy-5* and *Oxy-10, Persadox,* and *Quinalor*). Products containing salicylic acid may also be effective. The two other ingredients, sulfur and resorcinol, are often found in combination. These are weaker agents but may be helpful in mild cases. Avoid products that do not list at least one of the four active ingredients on the label.

Because each person's skin differs in sensitivity and each person's acne problem differs in magnitude, no single acne product is ideal for everyone. If your skin is sensitive and your acne mild, try a formulation that is milder than benzoyl peroxide—a sulfur/resorcinol or sulfur/salicylic acid combination. If your skin is less sensitive and your acne moderate, start with a benzoyl peroxide formulation. If the product seems unsuitable—too weak or too harsh—switch accordingly. It is important to follow directions carefully. If your skin becomes overly dry and scaly—even with a mild product—stop applications for a while and also cut down on your use of soap. If discomfort or scaliness persists, consult a physician.

Distrust the claims on an acne product's label or packaging. "An aid in the relief of acne pimples and blackheads," is

OTC acne products

CU's medical consultants urge you to read the label before you buy an acne preparation. The four OTC antiacne ingredients likely to be effective in the treatment of mild or moderate cases are benzoyl peroxide, salicylic acid, sulfur, and resorcinol. Product labels, however, do not always list the amount of each ingredient. CU's medical consultants have prepared the following guide to some OTC acne preparations on the market. Listings of these products are based on the presence of an effective ingredient in an adequate amount.

Benzoyl peroxide as chief active ingredient
　　Benoxyl (Stiefel)
　　Clearasil Antibacterial (Vicks)
　　Loroxide (Dermik)
　　Oxy-5 (Norcliff Thayer)
　　Oxy-10 (Norcliff Thayer)
　　Persadox (Texas)
　　Quinalor (Squibb)
　　Topex (Vicks)

Salicylic acid as chief active ingredient
　　Acnaveen (Cooper)
　　Acnesarb (C & M)
　　Acnotex (C & M)
　　Fostex (Westwood)
　　Listerex Golden (Warner-Lambert)
　　Listerex Herbal (Warner-Lambert)
　　Saligel (Stiefel)

Sulfur as chief active ingredient
　　Acne-Aid (Stiefel)
　　Finac (C & M)
　　Fostril (Westwood)
　　Liquinat (Texas)
　　Seale's Lotion (Dermik)

Thylox (Dent)
Transact (Westwood)
Xerac (Person & Cooly)

A combination of sulfur and resorcinol as chief active ingredients
Acnomel Cream (Smith, Kline & French)
Cenac (Central)
Clearasil Regular (Vicks)
Contrablem (Texas)
pHisoAc (Winthrop)
Resulin (Shieffelin)
Sulforcin (Texas)

---

printed on the label of *PropaPh,* even though the product contains no ingredients known to relieve acne. *Noxzema Skin Cream* claims to "help heal those blemishes for a clean, clear look." But it, too, contains none of the four ingredients most dermatologists agree are effective.

How informative are the ads? Not very. The medicine in *Stri-Dex Medicated Pads* "can get into your pores and kill bacteria that can cause skin infection." Maybe, but not deep enough to kill the bacteria deep in the follicle. *Clearasil* is "the most serious kind of blemish medicine you can get without a prescription," according to a television commercial. *Clearasil Regular* does contain a potent sulfur/resorcinol combination, but so do several other OTC antiacne aids.

Acne patients whose skin has not responded to OTC medications may decide to consult a physician. And certainly all those with severe cases of acne should seek medical help to prevent destruction of tissue and to minimize the possibility of permanent scarring. CU's medical consultants suggest, if you need medical help for your acne, that you first consult your family physician. Your doctor can then decide whether to treat your case or to refer you to a dermatologist. No physician can cure acne—only time can do that. But a doctor can prescribe medication specifically tailored to each patient's needs with dosage and proportion of ingredients adjusted individually. Acne usually can be kept under control until time obviates the need for treatment.

Antibiotics, in usual therapeutic dosages, have been prescribed by physicians to treat particularly severe cases of acne. In recent years, physicians have found that smaller doses of broad-spectrum antibiotics, administered daily for long periods of time (months or even years), have had a beneficial effect on many patients with moderate acne. This low-dose antibiotic therapy has been shown to reduce the concentration of free fatty acids that produce irritation. Acne researchers believe that antibiotics cause a decline in the amount of free fatty acids by decreasing the number of bacteria in the follicle, thereby limiting the amount of bacterial enzymes present. Many patients can safely continue low-dose antibiotic therapy under medical supervision for months or even years. Side effects from such use are generally minimal, barring allergic reactions. In the past few years, antibiotics in special lotion and gel forms have become available by prescription. They exert an effect almost equal to that achieved with oral antibiotics. This topical form of treatment has been beneficial particularly for those who suffer from side effects of oral antibiotics. For severe acne, benzoyl peroxide in a gel form and antibiotics—either oral or topical—are frequently used by dermatologists.

Tretinoin (vitamin A acid) was approved by the Food and Drug Administration (FDA) in 1972 as a topical preparation for prescription use only. However, patience is required; the acne may even appear to worsen during the first six weeks of treatment, and improvement is rarely seen before three months.

Central to the effective treatment of acne is the use of preparations that will clear the follicle orifice, thereby reducing the number of comedones. Tretinoin, available in gel, cream, and liquid forms, may be particularly useful in this regard. There has been, however, recent evidence that tretinoin increases the carcinogenic potential of ultraviolet radiation in certain laboratory animals. Persons using this medication should not only minimize their exposure to the sun, but also be under the continued supervision of a dermatologist.

In addition to the irritative changes caused by tretinoin, a few people may also experience a photosensitivity reaction (an intense reaction to sunlight resulting in skin reddening and painful blistering—see page 161) as well as mild loss of skin pigment. According to *The Medical Letter,* some clinicians believe that vitamin A acid therapy "represents an advance" in the treatment of acne.

Along with the new topical use of vitamin A acid, the taking of vitamin A in large doses by mouth has long had its advocates. In true vitamin A deficiency, the skin and the mucous membrane, including the lining of the hair follicle, become thickened and horny. Since with acne similar changes occur in the hair follicle, some doctors have reasoned that extra-large doses of vitamin A may prevent or cure acne. In most cases, however, the treatment has been unsuccessful. In one fairly large study, a group of college students with acne were given 100,000 units of vitamin A a day—about twenty times the recommended daily allowance. Slightly more than half of them showed some improvement—but so did half of a control group that received only a placebo. Taking vitamin A in doses greater than 50,000 units a day for several months has been followed in some people by loss of body hair, skin itching, enlargement of the liver and spleen, and a feeling of pressure inside the head. Such treatment is advocated by some authorities for short-term therapy in severe cases, but it needs close medical supervision.

One of the most promising hopes for acne patients was reported in *The New England Journal of Medicine* early in 1979. Gary L. Peck, M.D., of the Dermatology Division of the National Cancer Institute treated fourteen men and women suffering from severe acne with an oral analogue of vitamin A called 13-*cis*-retinoic acid. In thirteen out of the fourteen patients the results were dramatically beneficial in a matter of months. Side effects were minimal and not considered serious. Corroboration of those results may provide the medical profession with an effective antiacne drug in the near future.

The antiacne arsenal available to doctors also includes the injection of corticosteroids into acne cysts, cryotherapy (freezing technique), and incision and drainage of pustules. However, none of these treatments is yet capable of eliminating acne.

In treatment of acne, dermatologists recommend that the face be washed two or three times daily with soap and warm water. There is no actual proof that face washing helps. However, scrubbing with a soapy washcloth does remove some oils, dead skin, and surface bacteria. It also produces minor irritation, which may be of some help in mild acne.

In any case, CU's medical consultants do not believe that success in treatment depends on the type of soap used. Ordinary soap usually does an adequate job of cleansing the skin. Such heavily advertised cleansing products as *Noxzema Skin Cream, PHisoDerm Medicated Liquid,* and *Cuticura Medicated Soap* are no more useful than a bar of plain soap. "Acne soaps" with sulfur are not particularly helpful because the medication is likely to wash away with rinsing. Although some doctors may prefer tincture of green soap to ordinary soap, CU's medical consultants do not consider it of any special value.

Disregard the word "antibacterial" on the label of OTC acne products. While antibacterial soaps are indeed effective in reducing the number of skin surface bacteria, there are hazards in using these products (see page 144). Moreover, antibacterial soaps—which may be of some usefulness in certain areas (the armpits, for example)—are not at all relevant for acne therapy. Although bacteria are the source of the enzymes that break down oils into irritating free fatty acids, these bacteria live beneath the skin's surface, deep in the follicles. They cannot be reached by hexachlorophene (now available only by prescription) or by the antibacterial ingredients in OTC cleansing products. Advertising claims to the contrary are without basis.

Of limited value for certain people are abrasive soaps, such as *Brasivol* and *Pernox,* which contain irritating granules. These products physically induce inflammation, and can be quite harsh to sensitive skin.

Many women, influenced by cosmetic advertising, have developed the habit of using face creams in place of soap and water for cleansing the face. This is of dubious value for people with acne, because greases and creams encourage plugging of the pores. All so-called skin foods, skin tonics, lubricating creams, and vanishing creams should be avoided, too.

Even though the desire to cover up blemishes may be overwhelming, it's best not to use any cosmetics. For those who wish to use cosmetics, water-based products, applied lightly, are the least likely to cause complications. If the hair is naturally oily, it should be kept off the face. Although acne lesions do not occur in the scalp, hair dressings with a greasy or lanolin base should be avoided. Long-term use of such preparations can cause "pomade acne," a clustering of blackheads on the forehead and temples.

One of the prime temptations with acne is to squeeze and

pick at blackheads and plump pimples. Resist it. Handling acne blemishes can lead to secondary infections, rupture of follicle walls, and eventually to scars. The extent of scarring in acne, however, is not directly related to the severity of the case. It is the scarring potential of the skin that is the key factor. Although there are dermatologists who approve the home use of a blackhead extractor, CU's medical consultants advise against it because of the possibility of skin damage.

Since products containing iodides or bromides sometimes exacerbate existing acne or produce eruptions that look like acne, patients are warned against them during acne treatment. Certain drugs, such as cough medicines, sedatives, cold medications, and multivitamin/mineral combinations, may contain iodides. (Bromides have now been eliminated from OTC preparations, such as *Bromo Seltzer.*) Since iodides also occur in iodized salt, saltwater fish, shellfish, spinach, cabbage, lettuce, and artichokes, these foods should be avoided.

Most authorities agree that any other type of dietary manipulation usually makes no difference in the severity of acne vulgaris; at least one double-blind study supports such a hypothesis. With some people, however, it may seem that specific foods do aggravate the disease. The foods usually implicated in acne are sweets, nuts, chocolate, and fried foods. If any food seems to worsen the acne, try dropping it from your diet and observe the effect (if any). After a few weeks, reintroduce the food and again note the result. If the experiment convinces you that the food is suspect, try to avoid it completely. More likely you will find that changes in your diet make little difference and that you can eat what you like.

If careful trial of OTC medications (see table on pages 130–131) does not help, a physician should be consulted. Control of acne may not come with the first round of treatment. Those who consult a doctor for acne should be encouraged to be patient in following subsequent directions. It may help if you keep in mind that acne, which responds slowly to a physician's care, is likely to be even more stubborn with hit-or-miss self-medication.

While found predominantly in teenagers, acne is not at all uncommon in young and middle-aged adults, particularly women. Dermatologists who treat "adult acne" have found more often than not that patients in their twenties with adult acne did not have acne as teenagers. The abrupt onset of acne in middle age may be a symptom of an endocrine disorder, and merits consultation with a physician.

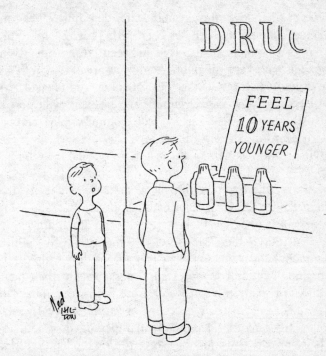

"But why would anybody *want* to feel ten years younger?"

11

Dandruff
and shampoos

Whatever their advocates say about new dandruff "cures" and medicinal shampoos, there has been little progress in the prevention or treatment of dandruff in recent years. Advertising campaigns have kept the public acutely aware of dandruff, and have promoted scores of remedies for actual and fancied scalp disorders. In a few cases claims have been so wild and so obviously false that the Federal Trade Commission has stepped in with cease-and-desist orders.

Oiliness and flakiness of the scalp are normal. The human scalp, even at its healthiest, shows a mild degree of scaling; the skin all over the body continually sloughs off bits of its dead outer layer. On the scalp, sebaceous glands add their oily secretion (sebum) to the dead skin scales, forming dandruff.

Most dandruff therefore is nothing more than this normal phenomenon, and a reasonably clean and healthy scalp can be maintained by shampooing several times a week with ordinary shampoo (or soap, in a soft water area). If there is much dirt in the air, or if there is excessive sweating, more frequent shampooing is in order. Even daily shampooing does not harm the hair or scalp. Brushing may serve to tidy the hair, but does not alleviate dandruff.

The main purpose in shampooing is to cleanse the hair of sebum, dead skin scales, and ordinary dirt. Obviously, it is better if the shampoo can cleanse without removing all the natural oils. Soap shampoos may be slightly more protective of the hair cuticle (outer coat) but may not cleanse as well as detergent brands, especially in hard water. To compensate for any possible harshness, various additives are used in detergent shampoos—for example, lanolin, which is purported to replace natural oils. Other additives are put in shampoos to meet special needs. "Low-pH," "nonalkaline," "pH-balanced" are catch-word phrases sometimes used by advertisers of over-the-counter (OTC) shampoos. The "pH" expresses acidity or alkalinity. A pH of 7 is neutral: Not acid, not alkaline. Acids with a low pH value will have a pH of 3 or 4. Values above 7 indicate alkalinity (hand soaps, for example, have a pH value of about 9). Because skin and hair are slightly on the acid side, makers of shampoos contend that a nonalkaline shampoo is less irritating to the skin, hair, and eyes. Laboratory tests have determined that most tested shampoos have pH values between 5 and 8. Consumers Union's chemists consider the difference between a pH of 5 and a pH of 8 too small to affect the hair or scalp one way or another. *Avon Protein Creme* shampoo, when evaluated by CU in 1976, had a pH of 9, which is less alkaline than a bar of *Ivory* soap.

Cream rinses may help neutralize the electric static charge in newly shampooed hair, thus preventing "fly-away" hair and making the hair easier to comb. People who think their hair could use more "body" may wish to use shampoos with protein conditioners that coat the hair to give it a thicker appearance. In CU's 1976 report on shampoos, panelists who tested shampoos rated *Protein 21 Dry, Breck Basic Texturizing with Protein,* and *Revlon Flex Balsam and Protein Concentrate* high on the list in performance for protein shampoos.

The precise cause of excessive scalp flaking is unknown. Sometimes the production of oily secretions and dead skin scales speeds up until the flaking is definitely excessive. But the transition from the normal to the abnormal state can be so gradual that it is difficult to tell when one condition ends and the other begins.

There is no basis for assuming, as some advertisers do, that germs are the primary cause of dandruff, and that an antiseptic shampoo is the cure. Indeed, although severe dandruff can be controlled, it cannot be cured. Spontaneous periods of improvement are common, a fact that casts doubt on all testimonials for cures with any particular product.

Dandruff is often confused with another scalp condition, seborrhea, in which there is an excessive amount of sebum. In the scalp this condition is characterized by very oily hair. It is common during the teenage years when the sebaceous glands are extremely active (see Chapter 10). When scalp redness and itching are associated with seborrhea, it is then called seborrheic dermatitis and requires a physician's attention. Frequently the forehead, nose, cheeks, and upper chest also are involved. The most effective shampoos for seborrheic dermatitis contain topical corticosteroids and can be obtained by prescription.

Selenium sulfide *(Selsun)* has been found to be effective in the control of excessive dandruff. It is available OTC in 1 percent concentration and by prescription in 2.5 percent concentration. In May 1979 newspapers reported possible carcinogenicity of selenium sulfide, based on the results of preliminary studies by the National Cancer Institute (NCI). Further tests are being conducted; the NCI's final conclusions will probably not be available until 1981. Meantime, CU's medical consultants advise dandruff sufferers to avoid the use of medicated shampoos containing selenium sulfide. Possible alternatives are available. Zinc pyrithione *(Flex, Head and Shoulders, Zincon),* coal tar extract *(Denorex, Tegrin),* and sulfur-salicylic combinations *(Sebulex)* all purport to have antidandruff properties. However, results with these and other products with similar claims may be variable and selection of a shampoo may have to be done on a trial-and-error basis.

There is no evidence that changes in diet or the addition of vitamins or minerals can control the development of dandruff or affect the quality of the hair in the slightest way. Nor is there any evidence that exposure of the scalp or head to sunlight either prevents or cures any type of scalp disorder.

Many men worry that dandruff might lead to baldness. Although severe dandruff and the male type of baldness (beginning at the temples and progressing to form a "widow's peak") may occur simultaneously, no cause-and-effect relationship between them has ever been shown. Dandruff and scalp oiliness can last for years without leading to the slightest thinning of the hair.

Most people who buy medicated shampoos fear being ostracized by a dandruff-free society, the creation of advertisers for antidandruff products. The fact is that the medical consequences of dandruff are few, if any. Although some dermatologists maintain that dandruff requires treatment, CU's medical consultants believe there is little evidence that scalp itching—the main symptom of dandruff—responds better to medicated shampoos than to ordinary shampoos.

12
Banishing body odor

Research has shown that sweat is not the culprit in the production of body odor. Rather, it is the interaction of sweat with the bacteria normally present on the skin that results in characteristic body odors. Two types of glands in the skin produce the secretions called sweat. However, normal secretions of both glands are odorless, or nearly so, until the secretions are decomposed by bacteria. The potential for odor formation is different for each gland.

The major source of body perspiration, the eccrine glands, are relatively unimportant in odor formation because eccrine sweat has only trace amounts of organic material on which bacteria can act: It is more than 99 percent water, less than 1 percent salt and other chemicals. These glands help primarily to regulate the body temperature and, for the most part, function to produce sweat in response to exercise, increases in environmental temperature, and fever. In certain areas of the body, such as the palms, soles, and axillae (underarms), they may become particularly active as the result of emotional stress.

Apocrine glands, in contrast, produce perspiration that is rich in organic material that can be readily decomposed by skin bacteria. Moreover, these glands, which respond *only* to emotional stimuli, are concentrated in the axillae, around the nipples, and in the genital area. The first and last of these regions are ideal sites for bacterial growth, not only because considerable perspiration occurs there but because moisture cannot readily evaporate. Apocrine glands become active at puberty. Although scientists believe these glands play some role in scent communication, their exact purpose is yet to be established. (Perhaps better understood than the biological function of the apocrine glands is their economic role: They help to support a $750 million-a-year industry.)

In view of what is known about the origin of body odor, there are three approaches that attempt to diminish or mask it: Replace body odor with another odor; decrease the number of skin bacteria; and reduce sweating.

The basic difference between deodorants and antiperspirants is that deodorants simply diminish odor; antiperspirants diminish sweat—and also decrease odor. The Food and Drug Administration (FDA) classifies antiperspirants as drugs because, by reducing sweating, their active ingredients affect a function of the body. Deodorants are considered cosmetics. But that's a fine distinction, since deodorants contain not only perfume, to mask the body odor, but also antimicrobial chemicals, to inhibit the odor-causing bacteria.

There can be little doubt that regular daily washing is the primary means of controlling both bacterial growth on the skin and body odor. The use of ordinary soap, which is mildly bactericidal, reduces odor by physically washing away bacteria and glandular secretions. Skin bacterial counts can be further reduced by daily use of soaps containing chemical antiseptics. But the routine use of antiseptic soaps will not prevent boils and other infections of the skin. Recurrent skin infections should be checked by a physician. They may be the first clue to an underlying disorder such as diabetes.

One controlled study demonstrated a statistically significant decrease in bacterial skin infections in users of soap containing hexachlorophene. But in 1972 the FDA announced that hexachlorophene would no longer be permitted in over-the-counter (OTC) preparations. An FDA committee of experts on antimicrobial drugs had recommended the action on the basis of data impugning the safety of hexachlorophene. Studies using both animals and humans had demonstrated that unregulated routine use of hexachlorophene could be considered unsafe. Microscopic abnormalities in brain tissue of newborns had apparently resulted from the absorption of this compound into the bloodstream through intact skin. Additional impetus to ban the antibacterial agent came after more than thirty babies in France died from the application of a talcum powder contaminated with substantial quantities of hexachlorophene. After the ruling on hexachlorophene, production and shipment of soaps that included it were halted; hexachlorophene products are now available only by prescription.

In 1974 the FDA advisory panel on antimicrobial products issued its report on antiseptic-containing soaps. Halogenated salicylanilides—the general class of chemicals used at that time in deodorant soaps—were recognized as potent photosensitizers (see page 161) and a ban was recommended against further marketing of these ingredients. Products have since been reformulated and now include other antimicrobials, such as triclocarban (used in *Coast, Dial, Safeguard,* and *Zest*) and triclosan (used in *Lifebuoy*). *Irish Spring* contains both.

These chemicals, like hexachlorophene, can be absorbed through the skin into the bloodstream. Animal toxicity has been noted with both triclocarban and triclosan. Although the panel indicated what it believed to be adequate safety margins, the amounts of these chemicals that can be safely used in a lifetime have not yet been established. Since safety and efficacy have not been conclusively demonstrated for deodorant soaps, Consumers Union's medical consultants suggest avoiding such products unless their use is advised by a physician.

Antiperspirants are relatively useless for a small group of people who have hyperhidrosis, an abnormality of the underarm sweat glands that results in the production of large amounts of fluid. At times this condition also affects sweat glands in the hands and feet. No entirely satisfactory solution is known for this rather embarrassing problem. It is thought to be due to localized overactivity of the sympathetic nervous system. Medications are usually of no help; in rare instances surgery may be required. Drysol, a somewhat more potent antiperspirant than those usually sold OTC, has been promoted as a treatment for hyperhidrosis. This product, available only by prescription, contains aluminum chloride in alcohol. Like other antiperspirants with aluminum chloride, it can irritate the skin and damage clothing (see page 149).

At times excessive sweating is an appropriate response to emotional stress or physical exercise. Excessive perspiration of the feet, however, may produce a particularly objectionable odor because of the action of bacteria on the superficial skin layers of the soles. In addition, retained sweat on the feet encourages the growth of fungi, which cause acute and chronic inflammations such as athlete's foot. People whose feet perspire excessively should, whenever possible, wear sandals or open-weave shoes, and hose of cotton or wool rather than nylon or silk. Liberal dusting of the feet with plain talc helps absorb sweat and discourages growth of fungi. Lamb's wool tucked between the toes keeps them apart and aids in the evaporation of perspiration.

In the past, some users of antiperspirants containing a zirconium salt (see page 177) developed granulomas—tiny, hard, painless, long-lasting lumps in the skin—in their armpits.

Based on data from animal studies, the FDA committee on antimicrobial drugs warned the agency about the possible dangers to the lungs from inhaling zirconium over a long period of time. Because this ingredient could pose a serious threat to consumers, the panel recommended that zirconium be prohibited from use in aerosol antiperspirants. The FDA adopted this recommendation in 1975.

Today's antiperspirants—which come in a baffling variety of shapes, sizes, aromas, and textures—all contain aluminum salts, usually aluminum chlorohydrate, as the active ingredient. In its final report, issued in October 1978, the FDA advisory panel on antiperspirants has also questioned the safety of aerosol antiperspirants containing aluminum salts: In effect, all aerosol antiperspirants now on the market. The panel has asked that manufacturers be required to conduct long-term inhalation tests to determine any possible hazards of their products' ingredients. Aerosol antiperspirants will be allowed to remain on the market pending the outcome of the tests—at least another five years, assuming the FDA does in fact require the safety testing recommended by the panel. The report suggested that pressurized aerosols pose a greater inhalation risk than either finger pumps or squeeze bottles.

The panel cited animal studies indicating that it may take years for inhaled aluminum chlorohydrate particles to be cleared from the lungs. In two other studies cited, aluminum chlorohydrate in aerosol form caused lung changes in animals. Both studies used heavy doses of aluminum chlorohydrate in a very small particle size, a size that increased the likelihood the chemical would reach the lungs. The inhalation studies suggested by the panel would more closely approximate exposure from normal human use.

The panel was much less concerned about nonaerosol antiperspirants. When applied directly to the skin, their metallic salts have virtually no chance of being absorbed or inhaled into the body. Local skin irritation can occur, but such reactions are neither serious nor frequent. Consumers Union's medical consultants suggest that if a rash or evidence of irritation appears, you should discontinue use of the antiperspirant immediately. If improvement doesn't occur within a few days, you should consult a physician.

It is clear—despite the ads—that no deodorant or antiperspirant is a substitute for washing. Some people who do not perspire much may find that regular bathing is all they need. Although soaps containing antiseptic agents can reduce the number of skin bacteria and thus possibly diminish body odor, it is possible to obtain longer-lasting protection against bacteria in the underarm area with a deodorant containing an antiseptic than with soap containing an antiseptic. More of the deodorant chemical remains on the skin compared with soap. In any case, CU's medical consultants are opposed to the use of antiseptic-containing soaps and deodorants—unless recommended by a physician—because of the possibility of an allergic reaction.

People whose main concern is wetness should probably select from among antiperspirant products. Antiperspirants are more similar than their advertising would make them seem. As Derwyn Phillips, president of the Gillette Co.'s personal care division, remarked: "The wetness-stopping properties in *Dry Idea* aren't any better than competing products. But the consumer thinks [it's] drier." This is not to say that all antiperspirants are equally effective. The FDA panel found, for example, that product type—aerosol, cream, liquid, lotion, roll-on, or stick—can affect the ability to reduce perspiration.

Manufacturers of antiperspirants evaluate how effectively their products reduce moisture by testing them on men and women. One armpit is treated with an antiperspirant, the other with the same formulation minus the active ingredient. An absorbent pad is then placed in each armpit for a specific time and the weights of the pads are later compared. If the pad in the antiperspirant-treated armpit comes out 20 percent lighter than the pad in the other armpit, the product is assumed to have reduced perspiration by 20 percent.

The FDA panel examined test results submitted by fifteen companies for sixty products. Aluminum chlorohydrate is the active ingredient most commonly found in antiperspirants. Products using aluminum chlorohydrate—*Arrid XX Extra Strength* roll-on, *Right Guard Powder Dry* aerosol, *Sure Super Dry* aerosol, *Tickle* roll-on, *Ultra Ban* lotion, among many others—reduced perspiration by 20 to 46 percent under test conditions.

The FDA found that test subjects could not tell which armpit had been treated with antiperspirant when perspiration was reduced by less than 20 percent. For that reason, the panel recommended that only antiperspirants proved by testing to be at least 20 percent effective should be allowed to remain on the market.

The panel also found that antiperspirant effectiveness varied with the product type. Aerosols were singled out by the panel as the least effective, reducing perspiration by only 20 to 33 percent. The panel suggested that certain inactive chemicals used in aerosol containers, such as chemicals added to prevent clogging of the spray nozzle, can impede the effectiveness of the active ingredient. The consumer, of course, pays extra for these inactive chemicals and for the propellant (about 80 percent by weight of the product), a sturdy can, elaborate packing methods, valve, and diptube.

Lotions were the most effective product type in reducing perspiration. Behind the lotions were the creams, the sticks, and the liquids. Roll-ons were the most variable.

The FDA panel found that *Certan-dri*, which contains aluminum chloride, was significantly more effective than other OTC products in inhibiting perspiration. But aluminum chloride is more likely to irritate the skin and discolor and corrode fabrics. The panel suggested that products containing aluminum chloride carry this label: "Warning—some users of this product will experience skin irritation."

Does putting more of the active ingredient in an antiperspirant make that product more effective? Products such as *Arrid XX Extra Strength* roll-on would have you believe the answer is yes. Not so, the panel concluded. A product's formulation—how the active ingredient is combined with the other materials in the product—apparently is the key factor rather than the amount of active ingredient used. If the FDA accepts the panel's conclusion on this point, extra-strength claims could no longer appear on antiperspirant labels.

There is one way that any antiperspirant can be made somewhat more effective: Apply it daily, well before its action is needed, perhaps as early as the night before. The panel found that antiperspirants are not effective immediately after being applied to the skin. Some become effective after a few hours, while others require more time and repeated applications to reach maximum effectiveness.

The modest reduction in perspiration attributed to many antiperspirants would not by itself be sufficient to reduce odor, the panel said. The panel concluded that antiperspirants reduce odor not because they reduce perspiration, but mainly because their metallic salts kill odor-producing bacteria on the skin.

A person may have to try several products until the most effective one is found. Although the active ingredients in most antiperspirants are quite similar, the FDA panel stressed that individual responses to different products can vary widely. But

CU suggests that, in shopping for an antiperspirant, the aerosols—particularly the pressurized variety—be avoided. Not only are they generally less effective but they also tend to cost more than the other types. And some doubts about their safety remain.

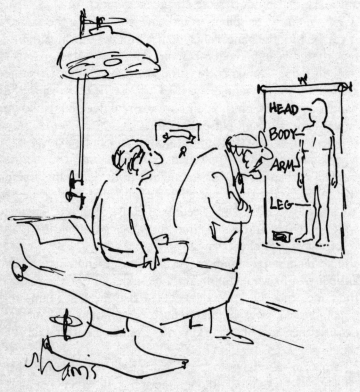

"Let's see now . . ."

Copyright © 1980 Sidney Harris

13

Products for sun worshipers

Suntan as a status symbol is a fairly recent phenomenon. For centuries the sun used to mark field hands and other outdoor laborers as members of the working class, while the rich treasured their fair skin. In the years following the industrial revolution, when the poor left the sun and grew pale in factories, a suntan gradually came to distinguish those who could afford the luxury of sun year-round. Despite warnings in recent years that excessive sun can damage the skin—and causes most skin cancer—a suntan may still be sought in some circles, but it cannot be justified on grounds of health. Skin cancer is most common in aging skin. Since excessive exposure to the sun's rays results in premature skin aging, skin cancer may appear in sun worshipers earlier than otherwise.

Although basking in the sun may improve the sunbather's sense of well-being, medical authorities recognize very few health benefits from such "activity." Acne and psoriasis are two skin diseases that seem to do better after exposure to the sun. Sunlight is also necessary for the production of vitamin D in the skin, although the amount of exposure needed is only minutes per day.

Sunburn is the symptom of immediate sun damage to the

skin. Although there is certainly a statistical basis for stating that more sandy-haired, light-skinned, blue-eyed people tend to experience this symptom than their dark-haired, olive-skinned, brown-eyed beachmates, the generalization may not hold for each individual. In checking the susceptibility to sunburn of volunteer subjects in a test of sunscreen products, Consumers Union found that dark-skinned individuals were not necessarily resistant to sunburn, and that freckled blonds were not invariably extra-vulnerable.

How long you can remain in the sun without being burned depends on the thickness of your skin and its melanin content. Melanin is a pigment produced by special skin cells called melanocytes. The number of melanocytes present in skin of people of all races is about the same but the ability of the melanocytes to produce melanin varies greatly and depends on an individual's heredity. It may also depend on whether you use a good sunscreen product.

The major problem with sunburn is the cumulative effect of chronic damage. Many fair-skinned people who are sun worshipers may develop wartlike growths (actinic keratoses) and skin cancer. Darker-complexioned individuals, whose genetic inheritance has enabled them to produce more melanin than the fair-skinned, tend to develop thick, leathery, wrinkled skin with a lower incidence of skin cancer appearing later in life. And those with even heavier deposits of melanin, as is the case with blacks, rarely develop skin cancer or other signs of chronic sun exposure. An advisory panel appointed by the Food and Drug Administration (FDA) has recommended that all sunscreen product labels state: "Overexposure to the sun may lead to premature aging of the skin and skin cancer. The liberal and regular use of this product may reduce the chance of premature aging of the skin and skin cancer."

Countless vacations have been spoiled by overenthusiastic

sunbathing on the first day. And the advent of the three-day weekend has brought more people than ever out into the sun, expecting to cram their suntanning into those precious few days. Even if fun in the sun is limited to weekends and vacations, most sunbathers can prevent both immediate agony and later unsightly peeling with judicious doses of caution and a good sunscreen preparation.

Both suntan and sunburn are caused by the invisible ultraviolet (UV) portion of the sun's spectrum. The amount of UV energy reaching a sunbather is affected by many things. The earth's atmosphere filters out some UV, so that a burn is more likely at higher altitudes where the atmosphere is thinner. This fact also explains why the sun's angle in the sky affects the burning potential; the skin burns fastest around midday (between 10:00 A.M. and 2:00 P.M.) and, some authorities believe, during the weeks just before and just after the summer solstice.

Other atmospheric conditions also affect the intensity of the UV rays that reach the skin. Because air pollution—a common ingredient in the skies of large urban centers—can obstruct passage of UV rays, sunbathing on the roof of a large city apartment building cannot be equated to sunbathing under the clear skies of a vacation spa. Similarly, haze and fog also filter out UV—but less than one might expect. Many sunbathers are badly burned on lightly overcast days when they mistakenly believe they are shaded from the sun.

And finally, UV rays, like visible light, are scattered by particles in the air, by light clouds, or by fog and are reflected from surrounding surfaces. Green grass and water reflect relatively little UV; white sand reflects about 20 percent, while fresh snow can reflect as much as 85 percent. In some circumstances reflected UV (supplemented by the refracted and diffused rays of the sun) can be intense enough to burn people with susceptible skin even when they sit for several hours under an umbrella or awning, sheltered from the direct sun.

The first time out in strong sun after a stretch indoors, you should be cautious. If you tend to burn fast and badly, the first exposure of unprotected skin is safest early in the morning or in late afternoon. Others can begin closer to midday but, for safety's sake, it is wise to spend no more than a quarter-hour in the sun the first time. On subsequent days, extend your exposure by quarter-hour increments. If you use an effective sunscreen, you can substantially prolong your safe time in the sun.

In practical terms, a person who usually gets red after twenty minutes in the sun should be able to stay in the sun for two hours (120 minutes) if he or she applies a sunscreen with a sun protection factor (SPF) rating of "6" ($6 \times 20 = 120$), provided the product is not washed or sweated off. Once a person's skin has become accustomed to the sun, a product with less protective capacity may be used. Specified by the FDA panel, the SPF rating (see table on facing page) began to appear on some product labels in late 1979.

Tanning cannot be rushed. Too much sun in too short a time only burns the skin. If you insist on tanning, the safest way is simply to go out into the sun every day and stay no longer than the maximum recommended time. For skins containing less melanin, tanning will remain an impossible dream. If you cannot tan, no product applied to the skin can help you tan, but a good sunscreen can decrease the extent of solar damage, i.e., wrinkles, actinic keratoses, skin cancer.

Before you place too much faith in any sunscreen, you should know that all such products contain chemicals to which a few people are sensitive. A new preparation should be applied first on a small area of the skin. If the skin does not redden or itch within twenty-four hours, there is little likelihood that an allergic reaction will occur. Nonetheless, use of any product should be halted immediately if the skin shows irritation, even if you have used the product safely before.

Almost all current commercial sunscreen products, whether sold as a lotion, cream, jelly, foam, or spray, contain chemicals that screen out skin-burning portions of the UV spectrum. But some products mistakenly used as sunburn preventives (baby oil, olive oil, cocoa butter, and mineral oil, for example) do not have any special screening properties. Such products do not offer any protection against sunburn.

Careful application of the sunscreen preparation to all areas of exposed skin is essential. Protection can be increased by heavier application of the product. But dermatologists warn

Skin types and recommended sun protection factor

Following is a numerical rating system for sunscreen users proposed by the FDA panel. Several manufacturers have reformulated their sunscreen products to reflect the panel's recommendations.

Skin type	Sunburn and tanning history	Recommended sun protection factor (SPF)
I	Always burns easily; never tans (sensitive)	15 or greater (ultra protection)
II	Always burns easily; tans minimally (sensitive)	8 to under 15 (maximum protection)
III	Burns moderately; tans gradually, to light brown (normal)	6 to under 8 (extra protection)
IV	Burns minimally; tans well, to moderate brown (normal)	4 to under 6 (moderate protection)
V	Rarely burns; tans profusely, to dark brown (insensitive)	2 to under 4 (minimum protection)

that if a greasy cream covers too much of the body surface at a time it could interfere with sweating, which could lead to heat stroke. Also, an oily or greasy preparation can lead to boils and aggravate some skin disorders by blocking the sweat or sebaceous glands.

Perspiration, swimming, and rubbing by sand, towels, or clothing tend to remove any sunscreen preparation; the film of cream or lotion must be replenished from time to time. And for maximum safety, the preparation should be reapplied after each swim or vigorous tennis match.

The suntan products currently on the market vary widely in their ability to protect against sunburn. (In 1971 CU tested thirty-three products, including lotions, creams, gels, butters, clear liquids, and aerosol foams; all screened out some UV, but none was judged to give everyone full protection to long exposure in the sun.) However, even the less effective screens are useful for people who are not too susceptible to burning and for those willing to limit their early exposure to the sun. If through experimentation you find a particular product works well for you, be sure to match the name exactly when you go to buy it again; many companies make several suntan products with similar names but dissimilar performances.

One group of sunscreens that merits serious consideration includes those employing aminobenzoic acid (PABA)—previously termed para-aminobenzoic acid—as the main ingredient. This family of sunscreens first came to wide attention in 1969 with publication of the results of a three-year study conducted by several researchers at the Harvard Medical School. More than 300 subjects were exposed to varying climatic conditions when covered with a wide variety of sunscreens, both laboratory-concocted and commercially available. Results showed that 5 percent PABA in 70 to 95 percent ethyl alcohol was distinctly superior to the other sunscreens tested, both in prevent-

Classification of sunscreen ingredients

The FDA panel has assigned classifications to sunscreen ingredients. You can check your sunscreen's ingredients with the list below.

Safe and effective
  Aminobenzoic acid
  Cinoxate
  Diethanolamine p-methoxycinnamate
  Digalloyl trioleate
  Dioxybenzone
  Ethyl 4-bis/(hydroxypropyl)/aminobenzoate
  2-Ethylhexyl 2-cyano-3, 3-diphenylacrylate
  Ethylhexyl-p-methoxycinnamate
  2-Ethylhexylsalicylate
  Glyceryl aminobenzoate
  Homosalate
  Lawsone with dihydroxyacetone
  Menthyl anthranilate
  Oxybenzone
  Padimate A
  Padimate O
  2-Phenylbenzimidazole-5-sulfonic acid
  Red petrolatum
  Sulisobenzone
  Titanium dioxide
  Triethanolamine salicylate

Not safe and effective
  2-Ethylhexyl 4-phenylbenzophenone-2 carboxylic acid
  3-(4-methylbenzylidene)-camphor
  Sodium 3,4-dimethylphenyl-glyoxylate

Needs further testing to establish safety and effectiveness
  Allantoin combined with aminobenzoic acid
  5-(3,3-Dimeth-1-2 norbornyliden) 3-penten-2-one
  Dipropylene glycol salicylate

ing sunburn and in resisting removal by swimming or excessive perspiration.

The Medical Letter has confirmed the value of PABA and has termed it "an excellent sunscreen" that can provide protection from sunburn and still resist loss of effectiveness through sweating. Commercial preparations using PABA include *Pabanol* and *PreSun.* These products cost about $4 for 4 ounces. It may be possible to save some money by having your pharmacist prepare a sunscreen based on a version of the commercial formulation: 5 percent PABA in a solution of 50 percent alcohol, 30 percent water, and 20 percent glycerine. CU's medical consultants suggest that you check the cost with your pharmacist; the price may vary, depending on the availability of some ingredients. Formulas based on chemical modifications of PABA are used in *Block Out* and *Sea & Ski* but do not offer as effective or as durable protection for the sunbather.

Another sunscreen of proven effectiveness is red petrolatum *(RVP),* an ointment now available over the counter (OTC) from Elder, the manufacturer of *Pabanol.* Of particular usefulness to those who may be sensitive to any of the commercial sunscreens are the products based on the "safe and effective" ingredients listed on page 157. These include *Uval* (contains sulisobenzone) and *Solbar* (contains dioxybenzone and oxybenzone); both products are available at drugstores. *The Medical Letter* warns, however, that some formulations are more vulnerable to sweat and bathing and presumably need to be reapplied more frequently.

For especially vulnerable areas, such as the nose and lips, a product that is a sunshade, rather than a sunscreen, may be necessary. Several OTC preparations are marketed for this purpose: *SunStick Lip Protection, Eclipse, PreSun, Uval Sun 'n Wind Stick;* but you can achieve the same result with a tube of zinc oxide available at drugstores.

Sun worshipers are targets for the promotion of less desirable products as well as useful ones. Perhaps the most curious of the sun-worshiper products are the chemical tanners that in 1960 became one of the hottest items in the drug trade. Dozens of manufacturers entered this field. The same tanning chemical, dihydroxyacetone (DHA), was used by all of them. Besides its use in straight tanning products, the chemical was added to aftershave lotions, sunscreens, and moisturizing creams. The profusion of products ended with the decline of the fad, but a few of them are still around. In fact, in 1972, *QT,* a sunless skin tanner, was the second leading product in sales of suntan preparations.

There is no doubt that DHA does darken the skin, but one cannot be sure the result will be the golden, natural-looking tan the products promise. Fortunately, if results are poor, the color wears off in a few days. In some users, the skin can temporarily take on a yellowish tinge; in others, the tan can be orange in color or blotchy. Also, DHA can discolor hair and clothing, especially with repeated use, and, as some users may have found out the hard way, the tan produced by DHA does not protect the skin against sunburn.

For those who insist on acquiring a tan without sun, there is a device more effective than chemical tanners—a sunlamp. However, it provides no health benefits for people with normal skin, is much more expensive, and may even be dangerous. UV exposure to the point of peeling may help in some cases of severe acne but should not be done without close physician supervision. A sunlamp may also be used in the treatment of people who have psoriasis. Medical supervision is necessary when a sunlamp is used to treat skin diseases.

The most immediate danger of sunlamps is the possibility of a bad burn. And just like sunburn, the full severity does not show up until several hours after exposure. Care should be taken not to exceed the time limits recommended by the sunlamp manufacturer. If users do not know how susceptible to UV burn they are, they should start with the shortest exposure time at the greatest distance recommended. Since it is not unusual to fall asleep while under a lamp, it is best to use a timer that automatically shuts off the lamp. Failing that, be sure to set a kitchen timer or an alarm clock.

A new sunlamp bulb may emit considerably more UV radiation than an old one. When starting out with a new bulb it would be wise to take shorter exposure times. It would also be wise to avoid taking hot showers or saunas before using a sunlamp. Drying off after a shower or a sauna removes some of the natural body oils that absorb UV rays, thus leaving the skin more sensitive to the effects of radiation.

The eyes need special protection from UV rays. Precautions should always be taken—even if the manufacturer of a particular sunlamp does not suggest any. UV can penetrate the skin of the eyelids and inflame the whites of the eyes; gross overexposure can even cause cataracts. Protective goggles must be used with sunlamps.

Anyone who spends much time in the sun ought to wear sunglasses. For maximum comfort the glasses should be dark, transmitting no more than about one-third of the visible light and, in bright sunlight, preferably no more than 15 to 20 percent. In addition, they should block most of the invisible infrared heat rays and the UV tanning rays, both of which in heavy doses cause eye discomfort.

The sunglass lenses should be free of distorting imperfections that can disturb the sharpness of vision or contribute to eye fatigue. A shopper will find it helpful to hold the lenses a foot or two in front of the eyes and focus through the lenses on some geometric pattern. The design as seen through the lenses should not appear distorted or warped, even when the lenses are moved an inch or two up and down and side to side. Judging from tests made by CU, a large number of sunglasses on the market has been deficient in this respect. Fortunately, less-than-perfect sunglasses are unlikely to harm the eyes, although they can cause eye discomfort or slight headaches with prolonged wearing.

Both plastic and glass lenses come in high quality, finely surfaced models and in inexpensive models with some surface ripples. Plastic lenses tend to scratch more easily than glass lenses, but they may be more protective against accidental flying debris. Most sunglass lenses are gray, green, or tan, although some are made in such colors as yellow, rose, or blue. The least distortion of traffic lights, or of any color tone, is with neutral lenses; CU tests found gray lenses the most neutral. No matter what color you choose, compare the two lenses to make sure they are equally dark.

Some high-fashion frames are so weirdly distorted that they allow too much light to filter in around the edges of the lenses. They also can be hazardous if they cut off peripheral vision. You can judge the quality of the frame by making sure there is no gap between the lens and the frame and no movement of the lens in the frame. The frame should have metal rather than plastic hinges with five or seven (not three) barrels and a screw fastener rather than a pin fastener.

Sometimes sun reflectors, widely advertised as an aid to year-round backyard tanning, also can prove hazardous to seekers of the sun. Dermatologists have warned that, if sun reflectors are used repeatedly for long periods of time, intensified UV rays can damage the skin.

A person using prescription drugs should check with a doctor before exposure to the sun or before using a sunlamp because a wide variety of drugs taken by mouth can cause increased vulnerability to UV radiation. Such a reaction is called photosensitization. The trouble could show up either as a burn or as an allergic skin reaction, and result in pain and severe discomfort from blistering. In some instances, blistering skin reactions have led to hospitalization; in such cases, patients sometimes have to avoid sunlight for indefinite periods. Less severe cases can be successfully treated with corticosteroids and temporary avoidance of sunlight. It is not unusual for reactions to occur even after three weeks have elapsed between initial contact with the photosensitizing agent and subsequent exposure to sunlight. With continued use of the causative medication, however, the incubation period can become much shorter.

Notable photosensitizing agents include certain broad-spectrum antibiotics (democycline, doxycycline, tetracycline), as well as a frequently used urinary antibiotic, nalidixic acid (Neg-Gram). Griseofulvin (Fulvicin), an oral antifungal agent, and certain diuretics, such as chlorothiazide (Diuril), also can photosensitize. One of the major tranquilizers, chlorpromazine (Thorazine), has similar capabilities.

Sunscreens, despite the protection they offer against sunburn, do not always prevent possible photosensitivity reactions caused by drugs. Different chemical agents, including the drugs named above, sensitize the skin to wavelengths in the UV spectrum other than those against which typical sunscreens protect.

14

Wounds, burns, stings, and bites

Normal skin is a rugged organ built to withstand considerable assault. Its mild acidity, oily coating, and horny outer layer of dead cells can protect the underlying living skin quite well. The skin's outer layer is subject to the constant erosive effect of day-to-day living, including bathing, scratching, rubbing, and other conscious and unconscious activities. These outer cells are continuously sloughed off, to be replaced in an orderly fashion by younger cells from the subepidermal layers. Thus the skin is a constantly self-renewing organ, ever changing, and not the static structure many people assume it to be.

So long as the outer layer is intact, most of the things—medicinal or otherwise—that reach the skin either intentionally or by accident cannot do it much damage. When this barrier is breached, however, as it is when there is a cut, scratch, rash, or other irritation, any topical preparation can penetrate more easily, with possibly damaging results.

Left alone, injured or inflamed skin has remarkable recuperative powers. Treated with the wrong chemical, it may find the double assault just too much and medication dermatitis may result. The skin may react with itching, redness, burning, rash, blisters, or even crusting or oozing. In some instances, additional self-treatment has led to reactions severe enough to result in hospitalization. The truth is that most skin ailments are better off without the many topical remedies found among the thousands of over-the-counter (OTC) preparations currently on the market.

Scratches, cuts, and abrasions

Scratches, cuts, and other small wounds can best be treated by cleansing with soap, thoroughly rinsing under running tap water, and covering with a small bandage for protection from additional contamination. Those who feel they must use an antiseptic should shun the highly promoted brand-name products, choosing instead isopropyl alcohol (70 percent), usually purchased as rubbing alcohol. Like most antiseptics, alcohol should be applied, if at all, on the intact skin around the wound, not in the wound.

The makers of branded antiseptic products do not share these views; indeed, in their advertising they often imply dire consequences if their products are not used. But whatever the advertisements and labels say, the truth is that first-aid antiseptic salves, sprays, and solutions probably do little good, and are rarely necessary. The impact of these products varies to some extent with the type and amount of active ingredients in each preparation's formula. The agents most commonly used in first-aid antiseptic products fall into several categories.

Alcohols. Most frequently isopropyl or ethyl alcohol is used. The former is much cheaper and just as effective. Isopropyl (70 percent) alcohol is probably as effective in killing most skin bacteria as any other type of germicide in common use. For first-aid use, alcohol is considered the most effective and least irritating of all antiseptics and is virtually devoid of allergic effects.

Tinctures (alcoholic solutions) are generally more effective than aqueous (water) solutions of a given germicide. But alcohol alone is as effective as an equal amount of many tinctures.

Antibiotics. Some antibiotic preparations intended for use on the skin are available without a doctor's prescription. Neomycin and bacitracin are the antibiotics most commonly used. A 1977 report to the Food and Drug Administration (FDA) —from an advisory panel on topical antibiotics—included the following opinion: "that no potential for harm exists when bacitracin is used on small wounds such as small cuts, abrasions, or burns." The panel recommended that use be restricted to small areas of application. Insofar as neomycin is concerned, the panel recommended that it should not be used in OTC medications labeled for treating large areas of the skin. Consumers Union's medical consultants, however, are of the opinion that the wisdom of using antibiotics without medical supervision is to be questioned (see Chapter 26). The overuse of topical antibiotics can lead to infections by resistant microorganisms, and allergic skin reactions are frequently reported, particularly with neomycin.

Bisphenols (bithionol, hexachlorophene). Bisphenols, if used consistently, are effective in reducing the number of bacteria on the intact skin surface, but they do not kill the bacteria as quickly or as completely as alcohol. In 1972 the FDA banned the use of hexachlorophene in OTC products in concentrations strong enough to be effective as an antiseptic (see page 144). Products that formerly relied on hexachlorophene—such as *Medi-Quik* and *Solarcaine*—have been reformulated using other antibacterials.

Halogens (principally iodine). These antiseptics are most often available as tinctures. Aqueous solutions of iodine compounds *(Betadine, Isodine)* currently enjoy great popularity. They cause less staining of the skin and less stinging and are almost as effective as tinctures for first-aid use; but they are more expensive. The iodine in these preparations can be absorbed even through intact skin, which can increase the blood iodide content. Although not harmful with occasional use, these antiseptic preparations can interfere with certain thyroid function tests.

Heavy-metal compounds (ammoniated mercury, phenylmercuric compounds, *Mercurochrome, Merthiolate,* and other mercurial compounds). Many are available both as tinctures and in aqueous solution. It has been shown that these compounds do not consistently kill bacteria with which they come in contact, although they may prevent these bacteria from actively multiplying. Allergic skin reactions may occur.

Phenols (carbolic acid, cresol). To be effective, phenol and phenol derivatives must be used in such high concentrations that they irritate the skin. Phenol itself is thought to penetrate the skin; if it does penetrate in sufficient quantity, systemic reactions, such as muscle tremors and convulsions, may occur. According to *The Pharmacological Basis of Therapeutics:* "Phenol has few legitimate uses as an antiseptic."

Quaternary ammonium compounds (chiefly, benzalkonium chloride). These substances are effective against the two broad classes of bacteria—Gram-positive organisms, including staphylococci, commonly the cause of skin infections, and Gram-negative bacteria, which also cause skin infections. The latter, however, tend to be more resistant and require longer exposure to the antiseptic. OTC products containing this class of antiseptic include *Bactine* and *Zephiran Chloride.*

Another product often found in home medicine cabinets is hydrogen peroxide in the usual 3 percent solution. Although it is a poor antiseptic, its frothing action may sometimes help to cleanse particularly dirty wounds.

"First-aid creams" are actively promoted as aids in healing wounds, but this should not be taken to mean that they *speed* healing. Very few data are available to show how effective they actually are. The FDA advisory panel, however, strongly urges the testing of these topical dosage formulations including gels, solutions, and lotions for possible OTC use.

The widespread belief that every break in the skin should be treated with an antiseptic results mainly from needless anxiety about the large number of bacteria normally present on the skin surface at all times. Most of these bacteria are harmless. Indeed, one school of thought maintains that such microorganisms aid in maintaining a healthy skin. The majority of organisms that enter a wound are handled most effectively not by an applied germicide but by the body's natural defenses.

These defenses, which are not fully understood, nearly always seem able to cope with the bacteria in a small wound. Certainly, one of the defenses is the physical barrier offered by the skin itself. At a wound site, the body must rely on white blood cells and serum factors, which become concentrated in that area. These defenses work best when the skin is damaged as little as possible, and when conditions in and around the wound are as unfavorable to bacterial growth as possible.

With this background, it is not difficult to outline a rational program for the treatment of minor wounds—comparatively small scratches, cuts, and abrasions. Three steps are involved: Cleansing the wound gently, cleansing the skin around the wound thoroughly, and protecting the wound from further contamination.

The cleansing of the wound itself should be gentle to avoid further injury, but foreign bodies—such as dirt and gravel—must be removed. Dead tissue and foreign matter in the wound provide an excellent medium for bacterial growth. Gentle scrubbing with a mild soap and water, followed by flushing with tap water, usually does a good job of cleansing the wound itself. Bits of foreign matter not removed this way should be lifted out as carefully as possible with tweezer tips wiped with alcohol. Spontaneous bleeding, because it helps to flush the wound, may be advantageous, particularly for superficial puncture wounds.

Organisms that still may remain after the cleansing can be eliminated by swabbing the skin around the wound with an antiseptic, preferably isopropyl (70 percent) alcohol. Within a few days a scab forms. Although not as effective a physical barrier as intact skin, it helps protect the wound during healing and should not be removed unless underlying infection is present.

If the wound becomes infected, yellowish pus will appear on the surface of the wound or under the scab. In that case, clean, warm, wet compresses should be applied several times daily. If there is no improvement, a physician should be consulted.

Some scabs are easily broken and additional protection is often advisable. A covering of sterile, unmedicated gauze and adhesive tape ordinarily suffices. Plastic adhesive tape, unless it is "breathable," is unsatisfactory in this respect. If the wound is more of a scrape than a cut, one of the plastic "nonstickable" coverings may be helpful because they usually do not stick to the wound. The bandage should not be airtight, since it might then trap moisture given off by the skin and encourage the growth of bacteria.

Small (less than one inch) lacerations will heal faster and with less scarring if the wound edges are brought together by two or three bridging pieces of tape. These are commonly known as "butterfly" bandages and can be made or purchased. Facial lacerations may require the judgment of a physician as to whether sutures will be necessary.

If the wound bleeds after a bandage is applied, and the

bandage becomes stuck, it is best to leave it on as long as the wound is healing normally. Pulling the scab loose when changing the dressing can only retard healing and increase the chances of infection. If a bandage must be removed, soaking it in warm water or hydrogen peroxide can help soften the point of attachment and make removal easier.

Do not try self-medication or home treatment of any kind if you have a deep puncture wound (because of the difficulty in cleansing it through the small break in the skin) or a large or badly lacerated wound (because of the danger of bacterial infection combined with the larger healing task confronting the body). Such wounds should be protected with a sterile dressing, and the patient should be taken promptly to a physician. Meantime, excessive bleeding from such wounds can usually be controlled by applying *firm* hand pressure over the wound (preferably using a clean cloth). *The use of a tourniquet is rarely necessary* and may result in irreversible damage to an affected limb.

One possible complication from any wound is tetanus (commonly known as lockjaw). People can best avoid this often fatal disease by being immunized against the bacterium that causes it. CU's medical consultants join with the U.S. Public Health Service (PHS) in urging that everyone who has not been immunized against tetanus take the full series of three injections of tetanus toxoid (the first two a month apart, and the third seven months after the second). After this initial immunization series —often completed in childhood—a booster injection is normally required only every ten years.

Even though an injured person has been fully immunized, a physician may decide that an additional booster is required. When past immunization appears inadequate, tetanus antitoxin (Hyper-Tet)—derived from *human,* not horse, serum— is usually administered along with the first injection of the three-part immunization schedule. Of course, the remaining two injections of tetanus toxoid should still be taken in the usual sequence.

Burns

Burns, one of the most common of skin wounds, call for special consideration. It has been reported that approximately 2 million burn cases occur annually in the United States. They are classified according to the depth of damage. In a first-degree burn, there is reddening of the skin, caused by the dilatation of small blood vessels near the skin surface. In a second-degree burn, serum or fluid escapes from these vessels into the outer layer of the skin, causing blisters. In a third-degree burn, the entire depth of the skin and some subcutaneous tissues are destroyed. Only first-degree and small second-degree burns can be safely treated at home.

The pain of such burns can be relieved by immediate immersion of the affected part in ice water or cold running water for five to ten minutes or longer. The procedure should be repeated for one hour with two-minute rest periods. Cold, wet compresses may also be useful as long as there is pain. This treatment, if resorted to immediately, not only soothes the pain but may also prevent blistering. A bandage, firmly applied, may also help. If blistering does occur, the dressing will guard against rupture of the blisters, as well as secondary infection.

There is no evidence that butter, lard, or cooking grease of any kind—if applied to the burn—is of any value at all. Vitamin E ointment has been promoted by some manufacturers as useful for treating superficial burns; CU's medical consultants know of no controlled studies to support the claim. Furthermore, its use may result in an allergic skin reaction.

Authorities on first aid and the treatment of burns agree that OTC burn ointments are seldom necessary. Most of these remedies contain one or more of the following: An anesthetic (usually benzocaine or lidocaine), an antiseptic, menthol, lanolin, cod-liver oil, and vitamins. Of these ingredients, lanolin, cod-liver oil, and vitamins have been shown to have no special pain-relieving value beyond that provided by petroleum jelly or similar vehicle in which they are contained. It also has been established that OTC burn ointments for preventing infection generally lack specificity and effectiveness, and in some instances may even interfere with healing. Furthermore, the anesthetic and antiseptic ingredients in some commercial burn ointments can cause allergic reactions.

Extensive burns (those involving either the face or more than just one or two small areas of the body), irrespective of their depth, should be considered emergencies and treated by a physician as soon as possible. It is hazardous to apply any ointment, oil, salve, or solution to a third-degree burn, because the drugs in the preparation can be more readily absorbed and cause toxic reactions. The depth of the burn allows ready absorption of any applied medication, for there is no protective skin barrier. Also, OTC burn preparations can interfere with later professional care.

Sunburn resembles an ordinary burn. If the sunburn is mild and without blistering, the pain may be relieved by compresses of cold water or by cool baths. Aspirin or acetaminophen in usual doses can help as well. Extensive sunburn or deep, blistered sunburn calls for medical treatment.

Stings and bites

People who continually scratch mosquito bites only aggravate the symptoms and may risk infection. Itching, which may be severe, can be eased by applications of very cold compresses (some prefer to soak the affected area in hot water).

Insect repellents can be effective against many insects. Fif-

172 The Medicine Show

teen insect repellents have been tested by the U.S. Environmental Protection Agency (EPA). The agency evaluated the technical data submitted to it by manufacturers and then made judgments on the products. Those that were judged both safe and effective are labeled with an EPA registration number and an EPA establishment number. The first number indicates that the product is effective against the insects listed on the label and is not harmful to people, animals, crops, or the environment when used according to label directions. The second number identifies the manufacturer. Some older products may still carry U.S. Department of Agriculture (USDA) numbers rather than EPA numbers; until late 1970, pesticide regulations were administered by the USDA. Look for EPA numbers to be sure the product is fairly fresh.

In 1977 CU reviewed fifteen brands of personal insect repellents and judged most effective those products using diethyltoluamide in the greatest concentration. Such products were found more likely to give longer-lasting protection against certain species of insects (not including stinging spiders, wasps, and bees), to feel a little less oily, and to be harder to rub off or wash off than brands based on ethylhexanediol. A product that contains diethyltoluamide will probably keep insects away, as long as they're insects that bite.

Some of the fifteen products contained a mixture of active ingredients. All the products included diethyltoluamide for broad-range protection. The other compounds included in the mixtures were, like ethylhexanediol, specifically effective against some of the insects listed on the products' label.

A repellent protects only areas that it covers. Except for eyes or lips and areas where there is a cut, bad sunburn, or rash, all exposed skin should be covered. Sheer clothing that an insistent insect could bite through needs repellent on it, too. (But read the label first. Some repellents can damage certain fabrics.) Pressurized sprays and foams containing fluorocarbons as a propellant are no longer available. If in doubt about a spray or foam repellent, buy a liquid, cream, lotion, towelette, or stick. These types of repellents are usually higher in active ingredients. All of the products carry a long list of warnings about where and how to apply them. Most mention the danger of ingestion and a few note the possibility of allergic reaction.

Stings from insects of the class Hymenoptera (bees, wasps, hornets) can be serious. A nonallergic person may experience various reactions, ranging from mild irritation and itching at the sting site to swelling of an entire extremity. Immediate treatment consists of removal of the stinger (should it remain) and application of very cold compresses. Anyone with serious symptoms from such a sting should see a physician. A few people are highly sensitive to the venom released by these insects and maybe are subject to anaphylactic reaction (see page 312), which can prove fatal. Such people can be made relatively immune with injections by an allergist. Obviously, they must be continually cautious and take protective measures against insect stings. Many physicians urge such people to carry injectable adrenaline (epinephrine) with them during spring and summer months. Portable kits containing syringe, needle, and adrenaline are presently available only by prescription.

In October 1978, a panel consisting of medical, legal, and public health experts addressed the question of whether insect-sting kits containing epinephrine should be sold over the counter. The panel concluded that OTC kits containing epinephrine should remain available by prescription only because of the possibility of misuse.

Bites by animals—domestic or wild—occur with some frequency, and because of the threat of rabies even a minor bite must receive careful attention. Although human rabies is rare in the United States, the Center for Disease Control reports that antirabies treatment is administered to about 30,000 Americans each year. Dogs and cats account for the majority of bites, but the most important sources of actual infection are wild animals such as skunks, foxes, coyotes, raccoons, and bats.

Even a scratch from a wild animal is grounds for a physician to consider initiating antirabies treatment. If the wild animal can be found and captured, it will be sacrificed and examined in a laboratory. The results of the laboratory tests are crucial to the decision about treatment. If the wild animal cannot be found and captured, the answers to the following questions will help the physician to decide the best course of treatment: Is rabies present in the community where the exposure occurred? If so, in which animals? What were the circumstances of the bite? Was the animal provoked?

For an extensive (or deep) bite from either a wild or domestic animal, a visit to a physician is mandatory. This is particularly true if the bite is on the face or neck because the incubation period for rabies is shorter at these sites. (The PHS reports that rabies treatment is rarely needed for bites of rabbits, squirrels, chipmunks, rats or mice because these animals are unlikely to be affected by the rabies virus.)

Dogs and cats that have bitten a human being must, if at all possible, be located and kept under observation for at least ten days. If the dog or cat is rabid, it will die within that period and its brain can be examined for evidence of rabies. Should the examination be positive, a course of antirabies treatment must be initiated at once. If the animal under observation remains well, no treatment for rabies is needed. If the domestic animal cannot be located, the physician will attempt to discover if the animal had been immunized against rabies and then recommend treatment after taking into consideration many of the same questions listed above.

15

Treating poison ivy

Poison ivy dermatitis—the rash that follows contact with poison ivy, poison oak, or poison sumac—is one of the most common of all allergic skin disorders. And for its treatment numerous kinds of over-the-counter (OTC) preparations have been introduced over the years. Unfortunately, there is no convincing evidence that any of these products is more effective than a few simple standard measures.

Although poison ivy dermatitis can be acquired in any season, the peak incidence occurs in the spring. The poisonous sap may reach susceptible skin not only through direct contact with the plant (or with its smoke, if burned) but by way of shoes, clothing, tools, and the fur of domestic animals. Such intermediaries, however, may be made harmless by washing them with soap or a detergent. The common belief that the dermatitis spreads as the blisters on the skin rupture is without scientific support. Only contact with the sap of the plants can cause the rash. One initial exposure to the plant is all that is necessary to set the stage for a potentially severe reaction after some future contact.

Sensitivity to poison ivy varies markedly among different people, and even in different periods of a person's life. In general, the degree of reactivity is highest in childhood and diminishes with age. It is extremely unwise to assume that you have natural immunity to poison ivy, since apparent resistance one year may be followed by explosive sensitivity the next year.

As a rule, poison ivy skin eruption appears one or two days after contact with the leaf sap, and the eruption can be unpleasant indeed. Anyone who has had a serious case, or has seen someone tormented with itching, will not be surprised that many potions and treatments have been proposed to prevent or treat this allergic reaction. Among the many agents at one time thought to be beneficial in relieving poison ivy eruption were bromine, kerosene, gunpowder, iodine, buttermilk, cream, and marshmallows, as well as a large number of botanical preparations.

Strong laundry soap has long enjoyed popularity. However, Albert M. Kligman, M.D., of the University of Pennsylvania School of Medicine, an authority on poison ivy dermatitis, has demonstrated that, in a highly sensitive person, washing delayed only five minutes after exposure does very little good; and in mildly sensitive people, the same is true of washing delayed for an hour. Under average field conditions, then, washing has little practical value. Similarly, little benefit is obtained from the use of tincture of green soap or other soaps based on alcohol or similar solvents. Once the rash appears, washing with soap may increase the irritation.

In general, barrier creams offer no protection against the dermatitis. Tests have proved that silicone creams, widely promoted about a decade ago, are valueless in preventing poison ivy dermatitis.

Kligman has conducted many tests with a galaxy of chemicals claimed to cure or prevent poison ivy dermatitis when applied to the skin after exposure or after the first blisters appear. Since poison ivy dermatitis is caused by a plant chemical, it seemed logical to try to neutralize this chemical with another. Many substances have been suggested, and many of them do indeed react with the chemical that causes poison ivy —but this does not mean they inactivate it. In fact, none of the chemicals tested had the desired effect. Kligman points out that, even if it were possible to inactivate the poison ivy material on the skin, the allergic process would start within an hour or two of contact, perhaps irreversibly.

One of the ineffective chemicals Kligman tested was zirconium, for which enthusiastic—and groundless—claims have been made. At least four OTC products used in the treatment of poison ivy dermatitis (including the popular *Rhuli Cream* and *Spray*) contain zirconium. Moreover, in addition to being ineffective, zirconium may be harmful. Even in minute quantities, this ingredient may cause granulomas—small, hard, painless lumps in the skin—in susceptible people. Granulomas may take as long as eight to ten weeks to develop following application of a zirconium-containing preparation, and many zirconium-sensitive individuals (and often their doctors) do not associate the appearance of granulomas with earlier use of a zirconium-containing poison ivy remedy (or at one time with an antiperspirant or deodorant—see Chapter 12).

For many years, physicians have used extracts of poison ivy, either orally or by injection, to build up immunity prior to exposure. *The Medical Letter* reported, however, that "oral hyposensitization with extracts of poison ivy, oak, or sumac is a tedious procedure with limited benefit and unpleasant adverse effects such as *pruritus ani* (itching at the anus)." Rashes and gastrointestinal disturbances also have been reported. Further, *The Medical Letter* reported: "Intramuscular injection of these antigens may cause unacceptably severe reactions." These include abscess, swelling and pain at the site of injection, itching, rash, and fever. (Insofar as antihistamines are concerned, they appear to have no value taken orally or in ointments and lotions, according to Kligman.) When the poison ivy eruption affects the face, genitals, or a large part of the body, corticosteroids (by mouth or by injection), administered by a physician, can be of considerable benefit. Such therapy is usually prescribed for only a week or two and therefore carries little potential for side effects (in contrast with external application of creams or ointments).

The widespread faith, even among some physicians, in poison ivy remedies that fail to stand up under controlled tests is probably a direct result of the fickle nature of the eruption. Its duration may vary markedly for no apparent reason, and the treatment being used generally gets the credit when the course is brief.

Most OTC products for poison ivy overmedicate. Almost all contain varying combinations of topical anesthetics, antihistamines, and antiseptics. Not only do these ingredients fail to relieve the discomfort of poison ivy, but they are also capable of adding to the discomfort by causing an allergic reaction. Consumers Union's medical consultants believe that none of these OTC combination preparations has been shown to be superior to ordinary calamine lotion. Therefore, they recommend that anyone with a mild case of poison ivy use the cheapest brand available of ordinary calamine lotion, apply compresses of cool tap water (although some prefer soaking the affected area in very hot water), and take aspirin or acetaminophen to help soothe the suffering.

16

Hay fever

In 1978 Americans spent more than $47 million for over-the-counter (OTC) products that promised relief from hay fever —the most common allergic malady in the United States.

Looking for the correct OTC hay fever remedy can be frustrating. Where to start? There are hundreds of nonprescription medications touted for this aggravating condition. And few are effective and medically rational: Some are too weak to work; some treat nonexisting symptoms; and some may do more harm than good.

Not every hay fever victim should be experimenting with OTC remedies. Some sufferers have what physicians call "perennial allergic rhinitis." They are sensitive to such substances as house dust, animal dander, and feathers, and their symptoms tend to last year-round. Because of ongoing symptoms in the nose and sinuses and the difficulty of distinguishing this condition from recurrent colds or sinus infections, people who frequently find themselves with sniffles should seek the help of a physician.

But most of the estimated 20 million hay fever sufferers in the United States have a seasonal form of the disease. At certain times of the year, a sensitivity to weed, grass, or tree pollen or mold spores (but, surprisingly, not to hay) brings on those familiar symptoms: The spasms of sneezing; the itchy, clogged, or runny nose; the itchy, red, watery eyes. These symptoms make it easy for most sufferers to diagnose themselves, especially if they know there's a family history of allergy.

Hay fever is something like a cold that lasts and lasts. But a cold is sometimes marked by fever; hay fever, despite its name, never is. A cold is not characterized by itchy eyes or nose; hay fever usually is. A cold can hit anyone at any age; hay fever seldom begins in anyone after middle age. A cold generally clears up within a week or so; hay fever usually lasts longer and will return, perhaps in milder or in more severe form, the same time next year.

Seasonal hay fever victims who find their symptoms incapacitating should consult a doctor. Those who suffer from mild symptoms, however, can try to ward off the allergy-producing substance (or substances) by installing an air conditioner or taking a well-timed vacation to a pollen-free area. If the first remedy isn't effective and the second is impossible, some comfort may be found in a carefully selected OTC remedy.

A panel of advisers sponsored by the Food and Drug Administration (FDA) made a three-year study of the safety and effectiveness of the ingredients in OTC cough, cold, and allergy products—including antihistamines and decongestants, which are used to treat hay fever. The tables on pages 181 and 185 list antihistamine and decongestant ingredients and dosages as recommended by the advisory panel in 1977 (and, in some instances, modified by the FDA).

Many hay fever products currently on the market do not meet the panel's recommended guidelines. (The regulatory process to change or eliminate such products could take years.) In searching for an OTC remedy, then, it's essential to read

Safe and effective antihistamines*

The antihistamines listed below were classified as safe and effective at the dosages indicated.

Antihistamine	Adult dosage

The following three antihistamines are alkylamines, *which tend to cause less drowsiness than most other antihistamines:*

Brompheniramine maleate	4 mg every 4–6 hr. (not to exceed 24 mg in 24 hr.)
Chlorpheniramine maleate	4 mg every 4–6 hr. (not to exceed 24 mg in 24 hr.)
Pheniramine maleate	12.5 to 25 mg every 4–6 hr. (not to exceed 150 mg in 24 hr.)

The following two antihistamines are ethylenediamines, *which tend to cause somewhat more drowsiness than those listed above:*

Pyrilamine maleate	25–50 mg every 6–8 hr. (not to exceed 200 mg in 24 hr.)
Thonzylamine hydrochloride	50–100 mg every 4–6 hr. (not to exceed 600 mg in 24 hr.)

The following antihistamine is an ethanolamine, *which tends to cause somewhat more drowsiness than those listed above:*

Doxylamine succinate	7.5 mg every 4–6 hr. (not to exceed 45 mg in 24 hr.)

The following antihistamine tends to have a stimulant effect rather than a sedative one:

Phenindamine tartrate	25 mg every 4–6 hr. (not to exceed 150 mg in 24 hr.)

*As proposed by the FDA Advisory Review Panel on OTC Cold, Cough, Allergy, Bronchodilator, and Antiasthmatic Products, with tentative modifications by the FDA.

labels carefully. That's especially necessary now, since manufacturers are in the process of changing their products to meet expected government regulations. A familiar allergy product may have entirely different ingredients by next month or next year.

Antihistamines are the mainstay of hay fever treatment, providing rapid temporary relief to most sufferers. Antihistamines act by inhibiting the actions of histamine, the substance that causes allergy symptoms. Some antihistamines also have a drying effect on nasal secretions.

Serious side effects are rare with antihistamine use in teenagers and adults, but drowsiness is a common complaint. For some people, that sedative quality makes antihistamine use undesirable when alertness is required, and potentially dangerous when driving a car or operating machinery.

Antihistamines depress the central nervous system, so the use of antihistamines along with other central nervous system depressants, such as alcoholic beverages, sedatives, and tranquilizers, can be hazardous.

Some people develop a tolerance to the drowsiness effect after using antihistamines for a while. And certain types of antihistamines are more likely than others to produce that side effect in the first place. Of the three main chemical classes of antihistamines listed in the table on page 181, the *alkylamines* generally have the least sedative effect and the *ethanolamines* the most. The *ethylenediamines* fall somewhere between. (*Phenindamine tartrate,* a compound with a different chemical structure from the others, commonly stimulates rather than sedates.)

While those chemical groupings can be used as a general guide, the side effects of antihistamines vary widely from one individual to the next. While one person might be literally knocked out by an alkylamine and function very well on an ethylenediamine, another person might react just the opposite. There may be need to experiment with different products in different chemical classes to find the most suitable one.

Curiously, children sometimes react to antihistamine use with insomnia and central nervous system stimulation rather than with drowsiness. Because of antihistamines' less predictable effects on children, anyone under twelve years of age should be given these drugs with caution—and probably under medical supervision. Children between six and twelve years of age who use antihistamines should take half the adult dosage. (Children under six, pregnant and lactating women, men with urinary problems, and people with asthma, glaucoma, or convulsive disorders should obtain medical advice about hay fever medication.)

Consumers Union's medical consultants suggest confining experimentation with OTC products to those containing one of the antihistamines listed in our table at its recommended dosage level. *Chlor-Trimeton Allergy Syrup, Chlor-Trimeton Allergy Tablets, Decapryn Syrup, Dimetane Elixir,* and *Dimetane Tablets* meet those ingredient and dosage requirements (see page 188).

Before making a purchase, ask a pharmacist whether or not any of the antihistamines listed in the table are available as a generic product. Buying an unbranded version may save you money.

Once a satisfactory antihistamine is found, it may be discovered that, after a while, the product no longer works. Just as it is possible to develop a tolerance to the drug's sedative quality, it is also possible to become tolerant to its therapeutic effect. Should that happen, a switch to another antihistamine could be in order.

Some currently marketed products combine relatively small doses of two antihistamines. But there is no proof that such combinations provide more relief—or even as much relief—as a single antihistamine in its full therapeutic dose. According to the FDA's advisory panel, such pairing of ingredients "would contribute to the likelihood of undesirable additive or synergistic effects. . . ." The panel recommends further testing of such combinations to allow for "the possibility, however unlikely," that they may have some advantages. Meanwhile, it would be wise to stick with a single-antihistamine product. Products that combine small doses of two antihistamines include *Allerest Timed Release Allergy Capsules, Allergesic Tablets,* and *Ginsopan Tablets.*

Antihistamines generally don't work well against nasal stuffiness, a common hay fever symptom. Some people are willing to live with their clogged noses as long as their other miseries have been relieved. But the less stoic long to breathe freely again and they turn to nasal decongestants to do the job. Nasal decongestants act by temporarily reducing the swelling of the mucous membrane lining of the nose. Some decongestants are available topically as nose drops, nasal sprays, or inhaled vapors. Others can be taken by mouth in pill, capsule, or liquid form.

According to CU's medical consultants, the topical decongestants should be used cautiously for hay fever because treatment is needed for so many weeks. Although the topical products work fast and deliver the medication right to the problem area, they can actually make things worse. Frequent use leads to "rebound congestion": The tissues swell more than ever as the initial effect wears off. Reaching for the decongestant again only sets up a vicious cycle that's hard to break. Topical nasal decongestants should *never* be used more than four times a day.

Oral decongestants are slower-acting, but they do not have that same rebound quality. And they can reach more of the affected areas through the blood supply. The FDA's advisory panel judged a number of oral decongestant ingredients to be safe and effective. They are listed in the table below together with their recommended dosages. *D-Feda Syrup, Novafed Liquid, Propadrine Tablets,* and *Sudafed Tablets* would meet the panel's guidelines. (Note that although *Sudafed Syrup* contains the same active ingredient as *Sudafed Tablets,* its directions for use would yield too low a dose to be effective.) Again, children between six and twelve who use these drugs should take half the adult dosage.

At the recommended low doses, oral decongestants cause minimal side effects. At higher doses, they can produce dizziness, nervousness, and sleeplessness. People with high blood pressure, heart disease, diabetes, or thyroid disease should consult a doctor before using them.

Safe and effective oral decongestants*

The decongestants listed below were classified as safe and effective at the dosages indicated.

Decongestant	Adult dosage
Phenylephrine hydrochloride	10 mg every 4 hr. (not to exceed 60 mg in 24 hr.)
Phenylpropanolamine preparations (bitartrate, hydrochloride, or maleate)	25 mg every 4 hr.** (not to exceed 150 mg in 24 hr.)
Pseudoephedrine preparations (hydrochloride or sulfate)	60 mg every 4 hr. (not to exceed 360 mg in 24 hr.)

*As proposed by the FDA Advisory Review Panel on OTC Cold, Cough, Allergy, Bronchodilator, and Antiasthmatic Products, with tentative modifications by the FDA.
**Based on phenylpropanolamine hydrochloride equivalent.

Because of the effect of oral decongestants on blood pressure, such products should not be used by anyone for more than seven days without consulting a physician.

Many hay fever sufferers use both decongestants and antihistamines. The two drugs can be taken separately or combined. Among combination products, *Allerest Allergy Tablets, A.R.M. Allergy Relief Medicine Tablets, Chlor-Trimeton Decongestant Tablets, Fedahist Syrup, Fedahist Tablets, Novafed A Liquid,* and *Novahistine Elixir* offer effective dosages of one recommended decongestant and one recommended antihistamine.

Such combination products are often more convenient to take than separate medications. But taking a fixed-combination product locks the sufferer into dosages that may not be exactly right. For example, a person might be able to get by on less antihistamine, and a reduction in dose might help in alleviating drowsiness. But cutting down on the antihistamine dose would mean also reducing the decongestant dose—and perhaps rendering it totally ineffective. And since a stuffy nose might not *always* accompany the other symptoms, a person who takes a combination product whenever hay fever flares up takes a medication for a nonexisting symptom. Because of such drawbacks, CU's medical consultants suggest using each medication separately at first.

Some cold and allergy products throw in an anticholinergic (a drying agent), such as atropine sulfate or belladonna alkaloids, to help dry up the secretions that produce a runny nose. But the effectiveness of these drying agents remains to be proven, according to the FDA panel. The agents were not classified as unsafe when taken orally, but they can produce dryness of the mouth, blurred vision, palpitations, difficulty in urinating, and other unwanted effects. The panel expressed particular concern about combining an antihistamine and an anticholinergic in a single product because of the possibility of increased side effects. Combination products with these potential drawbacks include *Contac Capsules, Extendac Extended-Action Capsules, Spantac Capsules,* and *Timed Cold Capsules.*

Another questionable component of some cold and hay fever remedies is caffeine. It's added, presumably, to reduce the sedating effect of the antihistamine. But there's no proof that the caffeine does counteract the drowsiness. CU's medical consultants believe there is no rational basis for including caffeine in hay fever products. Caffeine is a particularly unwise addition to products containing a decongestant, because both ingredients are heart stimulants. The following products contain caffeine along with a decongestant and should therefore be avoided: *Coryban-D Cold Capsules, Dristan Decongestant Tablets, Neo-Synephrine Compound Decongestant Cold Tablets,* and *Super Anahist Decongestant Tablets.*

A number of combination products also contain one or more painkillers, such as aspirin or acetaminophen. Some hay fever victims do sometimes suffer headaches, but a headache is rarely an ongoing symptom of hay fever, so regular use of aspirin or acetaminophen isn't necessary. Such use could mask the development of a fever, an indication of a possible bacterial or viral infection. A safer approach would be to take headache medication separately when needed. Combination products that contain painkillers include *Coricidin D Tablets, Coricidin Tablets, Dristan Decongestant Tablets, Neo-Synephrine Compound Decongestant Cold Tablets,* and *Super Anahist Decongestant Tablets.*

Aspirin poses an additional problem. Although allergic reactions to aspirin are uncommon, such sensitivity is more prevalent among people with long-standing nasal allergies than among the general population. Taking aspirin separately,

Hay fever remedies

The following OTC products contain safe and effective ingredients, in recommended dosages, for treating hay fever. There are likely to be more such products as drug manufacturers meet the recommendations of the FDA advisory panel. Products are listed by types and, within types, alphabetically. To judge a hay fever remedy not listed below, check its label for the recommended ingredients and dosages indicated in the tables on pages 181 and 185.

Antihistamines

Chlor-Trimeton Allergy Syrup (Schering Corp.). Contains chlorpheniramine maleate.

Chlor-Trimeton Allergy Tablets (Schering Corp.). Contains chlorpheniramine maleate.

Decapryn Syrup (Merrell-National Lab. Div., Richardson-Merrell Inc.). Contains doxylamine succinate.

Dimetane Elixir (A. H. Robins Co.). Contains brompheniramine maleate.

Dimetane Tablets (A. H. Robins Co.). Contains brompheniramine maleate.

Oral decongestants

D-Feda Syrup (Dooner Lab. Inc.). Contains pseudoephedrine hydrochloride.

Novafed Liquid (Dow Pharmaceuticals). Contains pseudoephedrine hydrochloride.

Propadrine Tablets (Merck Sharp & Dohme). Contains phenylpropanolamine.

Sudafed Tablets (Burroughs Wellcome Co.). Contains pseudoephedrine hydrochloride.

Antihistamine-decongestant combinations

Allerest Allergy Tablets (Pharmacraft Consumer Products Div., Pennwalt Corp.). Contains phenylpropanolamine hydrochloride and chlorpheniramine maleate. Met ingredient and dosage guidelines originally recommended by FDA advisory panel, and meets the modified dosage recommendation adopted by the FDA (25–37.5 mg of phenylpropanolamine hydrochloride every 4 hr.).

A.R.M. Allergy Relief Medicine Tablets (Menley & James Lab.). Contains phenylpropanolamine hydrochloride and chlorpheniramine maleate. Met ingredient and dosage guidelines originally recommended by FDA advisory panel and meets the modified dosage recommendation adopted by the FDA (25–37.5 mg of phenylpropanolamine hydrochloride every 4 hr.).

Chlor-Trimeton Decongestant Tablets (Schering Corp.). Contains pseudoephedrine sulfate and chlorpheniramine maleate.

Fedahist Syrup (Dooner Lab. Inc.). Contains pseudoephedrine hydrochloride and chlorpheniramine maleate.

Fedahist Tablets (Dooner Lab. Inc.). Contains pseudoephedrine hydrochloride and chlorpheniramine maleate.

Novafed A Liquid (Dow Pharmaceuticals). Contains pseudoephedrine hydrochloride and chlorpheniramine maleate.

Novahistine Elixir (Dow Pharmaceuticals). Contains phenylpropanolamine hydrochloride and chlorpheniramine maleate. Met ingredient and dosage guidelines originally recommended by FDA advisory panel and meets the modified dosage recommendation adopted by the FDA (25–37.5 mg of phenylpropanolamine hydrochloride every 4 hr.).

---

rather than in combination, would help in identifying the cause of any reaction that may occur.

Some people who are sensitive to aspirin also are sensitive to tartrazine (yellow dye No. 5). Although most of the tartrazine used in this country is added to foods, it's also present in approximately 60 percent of colored drug tablets. In susceptible individuals, it can lead to asthmatic reactions, hives, and itching. Even a low dose can produce a powerful reaction and can aggravate the basic allergic condition for which the tablets are taken.

In June 1979, the FDA decided that all OTC drugs containing tartrazine must list its inclusion on labels as of June 1980. On food labels, the inclusion of tartrazine must be listed as of July 1981. Meanwhile, people sensitive to aspirin or tartrazine should consult their physician about medication.

The heavily advertised "timed-release" or "sustained-action" cold and hay fever products should be avoided not only because of what's in them, but because of the way they work. Instead of lasting only three to six hours, the normal duration of drug action, their effects theoretically extend to eight to twelve hours. But "it's hard to know when the ingredients are actually released," according to Francis Lowell, M.D., head of the FDA's advisory panel. "The timing depends on a lot of factors in the intestinal tract. There is probably a lot of individual variation." If the ingredients are released too slowly, there may be no therapeutic effect. If they are released too quickly, side effects may increase in number and severity. Because timed-release formulations are not uniformly effective, the panel has recommended further evaluation of their safety and efficacy. The available sustained-action medications for treating hay fever include *Allerest Timed Release Allergy Capsules, Contac Capsules,* and *Dristan 12 Hour Nasal Decongestant Capsules.*

Of the vast selection of hay fever remedies lining drugstore and supermarket shelves, there may be one or two or a handful that can effectively and reliably relieve seasonal symptoms. Then again, there may be no OTC remedy that gives *sufficient* relief. Or there may be side effects as distressing as the original symptoms. If you are unsatisfied by the choice of nonprescription medications, consult a physician. A prescription product, or some other medical therapy such as desensitization, might prove to be a more appropriate treatment.

Even if a satisfactory OTC product is found, be on the alert for possible complications. Pain or popping sounds in the ear may indicate a problem that could lead to hearing loss. Pain above the teeth, in the cheeks, above the eyes, or on the side of the nose could indicate sinus infection, another possible offshoot of hay fever. Persistent coughing, difficulty in breathing, and wheezing may signal asthma, a more serious allergic ailment than hay fever. If any of these symptoms occur, see a physician.

17
Poison emergencies

A bottle of tranquilizers that's left out on the kitchen table . . . a safety cap not replaced properly on a container of drain cleaner . . . leftover weed killer poured into a wine bottle for convenient storage . . . a toxic houseplant left within range of a baby who's just learned how to crawl. These are just a sampling of the everyday situations that can serve as a prelude to poisoning.

Often, little harm is done. But some people become severely ill and require hospitalization. And some, ironically, are injured more by following the first-aid instructions on the package label than by the poison itself. As a cause of accidental death, poisonings are surpassed only by motor vehicle accidents, drownings, and burns. An estimated 5 million poisonings occur in the United States each year, resulting in more than 5,000 deaths.

Children younger than five are the most frequent victims of accidental poisonings. (Two year olds are at the greatest risk.) Curious, explorative, and unable to read label warnings, they may eagerly open a container of drain cleaner that's decorated with a smiling face, or a bottle of lemon-scented furniture polish that smells good enough to drink. Keeping notorious poisons, such as arsenic and cyanide, out of the house is not always enough to protect a child from poisoning. There are hundreds of thousands of potentially lethal household products readily available at neighborhood stores, and there may be more than two dozen such products on hand in the average household. The substances that most frequently cause fatal childhood poisonings are medicines, especially analgesics and mood-altering drugs, and petroleum products or other solvents, such as kerosene, gasoline, and turpentine. Consumers Union believes that responsible manufacturers of such products should be doing more to provide improved packaging and accurate label information in case of poison emergencies.

Poisoning deaths among young children are, fortunately, declining. From 1968 to 1977 (the last year for which statistics are available), they went down from 284 to 94. Most toxicologists attribute the decreased mortality to the increased use of child-resistant packaging and to educational efforts focused on preventing accidents in that age group. But among children over five and adults, the yearly mortality from accidental poisoning has almost doubled since 1968. Many poison control centers have, moreover, noted a recent increase in accidental ingestions of acetaminophen (*Tempra, Tylenol, Valadol,* etc.), an aspirin substitute. The proposal of the Consumer Product Safety Commission (CPSC) that acetaminophen be added to the list of products that must be dispensed in a safety container takes effect February 27, 1980. While safety packaging does lower the odds of a serious poisoning, it doesn't eliminate the hazard. "Fifteen ways to guard against poisoning" (page 200) describes some of the most important precautions to take for poison prevention.

As careful as people are about preventing poisonings, accidents happen. The first step in preparing for such an accident is to find out the telephone number of a local poison control center and to post that number by the telephone. There are about 650 of these centers across the country, most of them located in hospital emergency rooms. With up-to-date information on a wide variety of hazardous substances, the centers are able to dispense medically sound instructions quickly. To obtain the telephone number of a nearby center, look for a list of emergency numbers in the front section of the telephone book, or ask a physician, a nearby hospital, or the county or state health department.

Poison control centers vary in quality. If there's more than one local center, you would be wise to call in advance to ask about their services. For example, are they available twenty-four hours a day, seven days a week? Are the people who answer the telephones and dispense advice trained in emergency management of home poisoning episodes? Is a doctor available to the center for consultation at all times? Once the telephone check is complete, list the numbers of the centers by the telephone in order of your preference.

Another precaution that every household should take is to keep a bottle of syrup of ipecac, an emetic, on hand for emergency use. Available in a 1-ounce size without a prescription, syrup of ipecac is the most effective and safest home remedy for inducing vomiting. Most children will vomit within twenty minutes of its use, emptying their stomachs of substantial quantities of ingested poison. (Don't confuse syrup of ipecac with the fluid extract of ipecac, which is fourteen times more potent and highly toxic.) There are situations in which inducing vomiting would increase the threat to health rather than lower the risk of injury. Syrup of ipecac or any other method should never be used if the victim is groggy or dazed, has trouble swallowing, or is convulsing, because of the possibility of aspiration of the vomited material. If the ingested product is a corrosive acid, such as toilet-bowl or pool cleaner, or a corrosive alkali, such as drain cleaner, vomiting would cause additional damage to the esophagus and throat as the substance is regurgitated.

Although poison control experts agree that syrup of ipecac should be in every medicine cabinet, there's some disagreement about home use of another emergency remedy, activated charcoal. That black powder can bind a wide variety of potential poisons, making them unavailable for absorption into the bloodstream. Mixed with water, it's useful against such chemicals as antidepressants, arsenic, aspirin, barbiturates, and kerosene. Some critics point out that a charcoal mixture is messy to prepare, unappetizing to look at, and hard to coax children to take. But experience has shown that most children will drink it if it's offered in a firm, positive manner. If syrup of ipecac and activated charcoal are to be used together, vomiting should be induced with syrup of ipecac before the victim is given activated charcoal. Activated charcoal adsorbs syrup of ipecac and may reduce its effectiveness.

Activated charcoal should be purchased in powdered form. The pharmacist may have to place a special order for it. Research has shown that *AC-Merck, Norit A,* and *Nuchor C,* all powders, have a greater capacity for adsorbing poisons than do some other brands. In most poisonings, at least 30 to 50 grams of charcoal must be administered to adsorb the harmful chemical, so a minimum of 50 grams should be purchased. Activated charcoal is also sold as part of a mixture known as the "universal antidote," which includes magnesium oxide and tannic acid. In this case, more is not better. The charcoal may react with the other ingredients in the mixture, reducing the charcoal's capacity to bind the poison. Some toxicologists believe that the "universal antidote" is not only ineffective but dangerous because of the potential of large amounts of tannic acid to cause liver damage.

Yet another first-aid remedy advocated by some poison authorities is epsom salts, used as a laxative. But there is disagreement about its effectiveness in ridding the body of poisons—and concern about its safety. If not handled correctly, epsom salts can cause massive diarrhea and dehydration, especially in small children. CU's medical consultants believe it best to avoid use of epsom salts.

If it is suspected that someone in the household has been poisoned, what is *not* done can be as important as what *is* done.

- *Don't* administer a salt and water solution, particularly to a small child. Salt water is relatively ineffective as an emetic and potentially dangerous. If given repeatedly—as some label directions suggest—it can cause salt intoxication, seizures, and even death.

- *Don't* attempt to "neutralize" the ingested substance by, for example, giving fruit juice or vinegar after lye has been swallowed, or sodium bicarbonate, chalk, or soap after an acid has been swallowed. In the first case (an acid to neutralize an alkali), studies have shown that heat is produced, compounding the possibility of burn injury. In the second case (an alkali to neutralize an acid), carbon dioxide gas is released, which may distend the stomach and even cause it to rupture.

- *Don't* give the victim milk to dilute such fat-soluble poisons as camphor, phenol, or gasoline unless medically advised to do so. Some poison experts believe that milk, with its fat content, may actually increase the body's absorption of those substances, and that water is a safer choice.

- *Don't* give large quantities of any fluid, including water. One or two glasses of water may be appropriate for diluting the poison, but more than that may distend the stomach, allowing its contents to move rapidly ahead to the small intestine, which has a greater surface area than the stomach. So the

poison could be absorbed more quickly into the blood.
- *Don't* induce vomiting without medical advice. Although vomiting is often indicated, it can cause additional burns of the esophagus and throat if the ingested poison is corrosive.

It's easier to remember what *should* be done in case of poisoning, as outlined in "Dealing with poison emergencies" (page 203). Included is not only advice for ingested substances —the most common route for poisoning—but also for poisons that come into contact with the eyes or the skin, or are inhaled into the lungs. Whatever the type of poisoning, the most important thing is to act quickly, if possible even before symptoms occur. The idea is to dilute the poison and get it out of or off the body before it does too much damage.

When calling the poison control center, have the container of the poisonous substance handy so the product's name and other pertinent information is available for reference. And try to figure out how much has been taken, so a reasonable estimate can be given to the poison control staff. The amount of the substance swallowed may be a key factor in deciding if, and how, the victim should be treated.

Write down any directions for treatment and follow them exactly. Even instructions as simple as: Give the victim an additional glass of water. The instructions may be to induce vomiting with syrup of ipecac or, if that's not available, to tickle the back of the throat with your finger. When vomiting is induced, the victim's head should be lower than the hips to keep the vomited material from dripping back into the throat.

If it is not possible for treatment to be given in the home, instructions from the poison control center may be that the victim should be taken to a medical facility for evaluation and treatment. But even if the poisoning is mild enough to allow total home care and the victim seems well after treatment, it's a good idea to call a physician after the emergency and discuss the episode. A medical checkup may be warranted to make sure that no harm has been done.

In treating any poisoning, don't place much reliance on first-aid instructions on package labels. They're often old-fashioned and inaccurate and may increase the likelihood of serious or fatal injury. Some current labels reflect the state of the art twenty or thirty years back, when salt water was regarded as an ideal emetic, citrus juice a perfect antidote for an ingestion of lye, and chalk a marvelous remedy for an acid poisoning. But such approaches to poisoning treatment are now considered outmoded and potentially dangerous: For example, the common warning not to induce vomiting after ingesting petroleum distillates because of the possibility of getting oil into the lungs. If the petroleum product contains a highly toxic additive— such as parathion, an insecticide—vomiting may be necessary to get the poison out of the system as quickly as possible. And if the person treating the victim heeds the label warning instead of medical advice, the result could be fatal.

Some poison control physicians place the responsibility for solving the labeling problem with industry. A few businesses have come around, cooperating with poison control officials to devise accurate first-aid instructions. But the voluntary cooperation of every manufacturer of every hazardous substance is highly unlikely. Many companies have expressed the fear that a change in first-aid advice would be an admission that the previous advice was wrong, and that it would open them to liability suits.

In addition, accuracy in antidote information could hurt some products in the marketplace if competing products did not go along. Howard Mofenson, M.D., director of the Nassau County (New York) Medical Center Poison Control Center, gave this example: "If a drain cleaner label says 'No known antidote,' which is the true situation, and the advice on another drain cleaner is to give vinegar, a customer would choose to buy the product with the wrong label because it sounds safer. So no company in a competitive industry would want to be the first to introduce changes."

The response of government has been little better than that of industry. A number of different government agencies have responsibility for potentially poisonous products, and their approach is not always uniform. As a result, manufacturers have complained about conflicting rules and bureaucratic runarounds. Antiseptics are under the purview of one federal agency, disinfectants under another, and general household cleaning products under a third. There is little or no give-and-take among the agencies on the question of appropriate first-aid instructions.

The action being taken by individual agencies is painfully slow. The Environmental Protection Agency has begun a review of 1,500 active ingredients in 33,000 products under its jurisdiction. The process includes an evaluation of first-aid advice on labels of products in the most toxic category. But, according to an EPA official, the review will take ten to fifteen years to complete.

The CPSC, with responsibility for a large number of potentially poisonous household products, has so far approached the problem of first-aid labeling in a fragmentary fashion. Action began in 1977 in response to a petition by consumer advocate Herbert Denenberg to correct the labels on some 50,000 household products. In a small step forward, the commission revoked recommended first-aid advice for people who swallow alcohol-based antifreeze. The previous advice was to use a salt solution to induce vomiting, but "this instruction is no longer medically acceptable due to the danger of causing salt poisoning," according to a CPSC entry in the *Federal Register*.

That same *Federal Register* contained a proposed "Statement of Policy" by the CPSC to replace salt water with syrup of ipecac whenever the induction of vomiting is the appropriate first-aid measure. The proposal was made in July 1979 and could be in effect by the end of 1979.

In January 1978, CU warned that some first-aid instructions on the labels of household poisons could actually increase the likelihood of serious or fatal injury because the instructions were out of date or inaccurate. We called for the creation of a committee of experts to recommend government policy and regulations to straighten out the jumble of poison-control instructions. In the fall of 1978, partially in response to our plea, Congress established the Toxicological Advisory Board. The purpose of this nine-member panel, which will exist for four years, is to review the CPSC's existing guidelines and to recommend changes in labeling and poison antidotes.

Along these lines, the National Poison Control Network has petitioned the Food and Drug Administration to require labels warning patients of the hazards of overmedication on all over-the-counter drug products. An overdose statement, simple enough to be read by a person with an eighth-grade education, should be used. The following has been proposed: "Read This First: The directions on this package tell you how much and how often to take this medicine. Taking more can hurt you. This is true of all drugs. If you think someone has taken too much, call your poison center, hospital emergency room or doctor now. Keep this and all medicines away from children."

Fifteen ways to guard against poisoning

Any poisoning emergency can be a severely traumatic event, especially for a child. Prevention is vastly preferable to undergoing such a frightening and often painful experience. By buying, storing, using, and discarding products with care, a poisoning can be prevented. Although some of these suggestions are most relevant to households with small children, an awareness of poison-prevention principles can help to make any home safer.

1. If a medicine or other product is available in child-resistant packaging, buy it that way—even if it also comes in a more convenient or economical size in an easy-to-open container. (If, on the other hand, child-resistant containers are difficult to open because of a disability and there are no young children in the home, buy regular packaging. By law, every product available with safety lids can also be packaged in one size without them. And any physician or patient can request non-safety packaging for prescription medication.)

2. Try to see any potentially dangerous product as a child would. Does the package or its contents have an appealing color or shape? Does a pretty picture decorate the label? Is the product lemon-scented, or candy-coated, or is it otherwise appealing in smell or taste? If so, find a less attractive substitute. (CU has, for many years, warned against the use of flavored aspirin for children—see page 31 for CU's advice on how best to give aspirin to children.)

3. Where possible, select the safest product for a particular need. For example, instead of bringing home a chemical drain cleaner, try using a rubber plunger and "snake" or drain auger. In place of a toilet-bowl cleaner, use a brush and a general-purpose household cleaner. It may be possible to do without camphorated oil, oil of wintergreen, boric acid, rat and insect poisons. Such common poisonous plants as philodendrons, castor beans, rosary peas, daffodils, and hyacinths are best not bought or grown in the home.

4. If a highly toxic substance must be purchased to perform a particular function, buy only enough for that job.

5. Keep medicines, household cleaning products, and other

potentially hazardous substances out of the reach of children. Preferably, these products should be locked up, or kept in a cabinet with a child-protection latch (available at hardware stores). As an added safeguard, some parents mark toxic products with stickers of cartoon characters, such as Mr. Yuk or Officer Ugg and his Poison Patrol, to help children identify and avoid those substances.

6. All potentially poisonous products should be kept in their original container with the label intact. Toxic substances should never be placed in food containers. Adults as well as children have been poisoned as a result of such switches.

7. If a cleaning product looks similar to a food product, don't keep them side by side. Otherwise, a child thirsting for some soda or juice may down a swig of furniture polish instead.

8. Make sure that all medicines are clearly labeled. Don't keep them near foods, and don't leave them carelessly in a purse, jacket pocket, or bureau drawer.

9. Read the safety warnings printed on the package label before using a product and follow those directions closely.

10. Never take pills in front of a small child; youngsters are inveterate imitators. And *never* refer to the pills given to children as "candy."

11. Don't leave a hazardous product unguarded while it is in use. Many childhood poisonings occur when an adult is called away to answer a doorbell or telephone and a child is left alone with a poisonous substance.

12. Work with household chemicals in a well-ventilated area. Some of them give off fumes that may be dangerous at high concentrations. And some, such as chlorine bleach and ammonia, are incompatible; they may produce toxic gases if mixed together.

13. Replace safety lids properly right after use and put the product away.

14. Dispose of the remainder of any potentially poisonous material after the product has done its job.

15. Whenever possible, dispose of the toxic substance by pouring it down a drain or flushing it down a toilet. And don't forget about the container. It may still have enough dangerous material left inside to do damage. Make sure to rinse out the container carefully before throwing it away.

Dealing with poison emergencies

Despite the best preventive efforts, poisonings can still happen. Most commonly, they will be the result of swallowing of household products. They can also result from the accidental spilling of a poison, which can damage the eyes and the skin. And the inhalation of a poison can cause respiratory failure.

Swallowed poisons. If the victim is conscious and can swallow, immediately give a glass or two of water. Then call a poison control center. If one can't be reached, call a physician or a hospital emergency room. If the advice you are given conflicts with that on the product's label, ignore the label—its first-aid instructions may be based on outdated information.

If the victim is *convulsing,* immediately call an ambulance or the police. While waiting for help, cradle the person's head in your arms and try to keep the neck extended back to keep the airway open. Also try to put a small soft cloth between the teeth to prevent biting of the tongue. Do not attempt to restrict the arm and leg movements; gentle restraint to avoid bodily harm against walls or furniture is all that is necessary.

If the victim is unusually *drowsy* or *unconscious,* call an ambulance or the police at once. Meanwhile, lay the victim flat with a small pillow or rolled towel under the neck to help keep the airway open, and position the head to one side to prevent any vomited material from getting into the lungs.

Poisons in the eye. Immediately wash the eye with lukewarm water for at least fifteen minutes. The water should be running in a stream across the eye, and the eyelid should be held open so the poison is not trapped underneath it. The time it may take to travel to a hospital before washing the eye could permanently damage the cornea. It is important to take the time to flush the eye immediately, even before calling a poison control center, physician, or emergency health facility.

Poisons on the skin. Take off any affected clothing. If solid particles of the poisonous material are left on the skin or in the hair, remove them with a cloth or paper towel to avoid further damage. Then flush the skin area with lukewarm water for at least fifteen minutes, perhaps by means of a long shower. Once that procedure is completed, call a poison control center, doctor, or emergency room.

Inhaled poisons. Immediately move the victim from the contaminated area into fresh air, but be sure to avoid exposure to the vapor. (One method of protection is to put a wet towel over your face while moving the victim.) If breathing or heart beat has stopped, at once begin cardiopulmonary resuscitation (CPR). If anyone else is present while CPR is being applied, ask that person to call for medical help and ask that an oxygen supply be brought along. (Courses in CPR are given regularly in many communities. Inquire at the local fire, police, or volunteer ambulance departments. Community hospitals, American Red Cross, and the County Medical Society may also provide information on CPR training courses.)

18

Women and iron

Physicians of ancient times would dip a sword into water and have a patient drink the liquid to absorb the strength of the sword's iron. They may have derived the therapy from the myth of Iphyelus, who was cured of impotence by drinking iron rust dissolved in wine.

Medicine has taken great strides since those days, and so have those who sell iron as a restorative. By the mid-1940s, Americans were being warned in advertisements of the perils of "tired blood"; iron-containing *Geritol,* people were told, would restore lost vitality.

Today, the target of the ads is more specific: women. One *Geritol* ad campaign, for example, depicts women who "take good care" of themselves by exercising, eating right—and taking *Geritol.* Adoring husbands then reward them with a kiss for such healthful habits. Another *Geritol* television commercial shows a woman who takes the preparation "to look as young as I can." A commercial for *One a Day Plus Iron* presents the product as a way to get enough iron without overeating. And a magazine ad for *Stresstabs 600 With Iron* refers to the mineral as "a touch of womanhood."

Such promotional claims make the most of a good thing.

Iron is essential to life. It's a key component of hemoglobin, the protein in blood that transports oxygen to the cells. It is also a constituent of muscle protein and of several enzymes that allow cells to convert nutrients into energy.

It's a fact that iron deficiency is a common nutritional disorder. It occurs when iron losses from the body—usually from some form of bleeding—exceed the amounts of iron ingested in the ordinary diet. The body then draws on its iron stores in the liver, spleen, and bone marrow. But, in time, these reserves become depleted. Next, the production of red blood cells in the bone marrow is impaired. Finally, continued lack of iron results in iron-deficiency anemia. Shortchanged of hemoglobin, the red blood cells become smaller and paler than normal, and the delivery of oxygen to the tissues is compromised.

Although most iron supplements are not promoted as cures for iron-deficiency anemia, there is at least one irresponsible exception. A magazine ad for *Geritol* refers to "iron-poor blood" (a slight switch from the "tired" variety), and claims that "*Geritol*'s iron will actually build your blood back to normal." But anyone whose blood is not "normal" should be under a physician's care, not under the care of commercial hucksters. Treatment of iron-deficiency anemia requires *therapeutic* doses of iron, which are larger than the supplemental doses used to offset a marginal diet.

Self-diagnosis, moreover, is a tricky business. Weakness, listlessness, and the tendency to tire easily can signal a number of conditions other than anemia. Furthermore, all anemias are not due to iron deficiency. Some are caused by red blood cell destruction, bone marrow failure, or deficiencies of other nutrients necessary for red blood cell production, such as vitamin B_{12} and folic acid. Many anemic people are without symptoms and haven't a clue to their anemia until a routine blood test uncovers a low blood count (less hemoglobin and a lower number of red blood cells than normal). People with mild anemia generally don't feel sick and show little or no apparent evidence of harm.

People who suffer from severe anemia often have symptoms, such as palpitations, headache, difficulty in breathing during exertion, extreme tiredness, and pallor. Anyone with such symptoms should seek medical help, not an advertised elixir. Appropriate treatment is important because severe anemia can lead to poor function of several vital organs, including the heart and brain. When anemia develops rapidly, as in acute blood loss, the symptoms are usually marked and a transfusion may be necessary. Conversely, when anemia develops gradually over a long period, the body compensates in various ways and symptoms may be absent or minimal. The treatment regimen for mild iron-deficiency anemia generally involves a few months of taking iron pills, in the correct dosage, several times a day.

But what if you feel just fine but are bombarded by television commercials suggesting that you take a daily iron supplement? Are you really a likely candidate for iron-deficiency anemia? And, if you are, what should you do about it?

For men and for women past menopause, iron supplementation is generally unnecessary and potentially harmful. A normal diet provides quite enough iron. To offset normal iron losses, adult men and postmenopausal women need about 10 milligrams (mg) of iron a day, according to the Recommended Daily Allowances (RDA) set by the National Academy of Sciences–National Research Council. The average adult diet in the United States provides about 6 mg of iron for each 1,000 calories, or about 10 to 20 mg a day. So any added iron in the form of an advertised supplement is usually a waste of money.

Iron deficiency in men and postmenopausal women is almost always due to abnormal and persistent blood loss rather than to poor diet. The cause of the bleeding may be an ulcer, stomach irritation from excessive aspirin or alcohol usage, a polyp of the intestine, or even hemorrhoids. It might also be a sign of cancer somewhere in the gastrointestinal tract. In fact, iron-deficiency anemia may be the first indication of colon cancer, and discovering the anemia can lead to early diagnosis of such cancer in a curable stage. But self-medication with iron that delays or prevents the development of anemia can obscure the diagnosis and hamper optimum treatment of the malignancy. Iron also causes blackening of the stools, which may mask a similar discoloration resulting from intestinal bleeding.

Another possible danger of supplementation is iron overload, especially in people who can't regulate iron absorption properly. Overload is not common, but it can be harmful when it does occur, damaging the liver, pancreas, or heart.

Most advertising for iron supplements is directed to premenopausal women, an audience less likely to be harmed. But some promotions have a general appeal. The *Geritol* ad discussing "iron-poor blood," for example, has appeared in such family publications as *Reader's Digest* and the New York *Daily News.* The copy makes no attempt to exclude either sex or any age group from its advertising message. And the *Geritol* commercial depicting a woman who knows she's "not getting any younger" makes a deliberate appeal to older women.

There are some groups in the population that may need more iron than is available in their diet. Population studies have uncovered a high prevalence of iron-deficiency anemia in children from six months to five years of age. Young children have high iron needs because of their rapid growth and expanding blood volume.

Many pediatricians recommend iron-enriched foods to meet the additional iron requirement. Some prescribe iron supplements. In fact, an advisory panel on Over-the-Counter (OTC) Vitamin and Mineral Drug Products has recommended to the

Food and Drug Administration (FDA) that OTC drug products containing 10 to 15 mg of iron be made available for young children. But the panel's report stresses that the need for any vitamin or mineral therapy should be determined by a physician.

Pregnant women also tend to need more iron than their diet provides. During the latter half of pregnancy, about 500 to 700 mg of iron are transferred to the growing fetus and placenta. But the average woman has only about 300 mg of iron stored up. So she is more likely than not to become iron-deficient during pregnancy. The FDA advisory panel recommended that an OTC tablet containing 30 to 60 mg of iron be made available for pregnant women to prevent iron deficiency. As part of good prenatal care, pregnant women should receive advice on iron supplementation from their physicians.

The most difficult decision about iron supplements falls to the nonpregnant woman of childbearing age. She may not be getting enough iron from her food to make up for the loss of iron during menstrual bleeding. The chances are about one in ten that she has iron-deficiency anemia, and about three in ten that she has insufficient iron stores to see her through a pregnancy or a few episodes of heavy menstrual bleeding.

The RDA for iron in menstruating women is 18 mg. But women get only 9 to 12 mg, on average, from a balanced diet. The ads for iron supplements take full advantage of that discrepancy. According to a television commercial for *One a Day Plus Iron,* to get enough iron "you'd probably have to overeat. And that's not good. So many of you may not get enough. That's not good either." What's good? *One a Day Plus Iron,* naturally. An ad for *FemIron* shows a smiling young woman who "may look healthy, but like most young women, she probably doesn't get enough of the iron that's vital to good health." And so, the ad continues, "That's why there's *FemIron.*"

One nationwide survey found that 95 percent of women of childbearing age *don't* get the recommended amount of iron. How, then, do most women manage to avoid iron deficiency? Apparently, the RDA of 18 mg *exceeds* the needs of most women. RDAs are recommendations for *groups* of people, not individuals, and are set with the idea of meeting the needs of nearly the entire population, including people who require more than the average. Accordingly, the RDAs generally contain a substantial cushion, or "margin of sufficiency," above the requirements of the average individual. In fact, one study suggests that a daily iron intake of 11 to 12 mg may be sufficient to prevent iron deficiency in most menstruating women.

How can a woman tell if she's at risk of becoming iron deficient? The most revealing clue is the amount of blood lost each month as part of the menstrual flow. Excessive loss of blood means excessive loss of iron, and roughly one woman in ten experiences profuse menstrual flow. A woman should consider her flow excessive if:

- She finds it necessary to use both tampons and pads during the first two or three days of her menstrual period.
- The pads are soaked through every hour or two toward the beginning of a period.
- The flow includes clots, especially clots of an inch or so in diameter or clots that persist after the first day.
- The menstrual blood flow lasts more than seven days.

Birth control practices can be a factor in blood flow. Oral contraceptive pills tend to reduce monthly blood loss, while intrauterine devices generally produce an increase. One study showed that the loss of blood doubled in a group of twenty women after intrauterine devices were inserted.

Meats (especially liver), fish, green leafy vegetables, beans, dried fruits, and whole wheat are all rich in iron. But the body absorbs only about 5 percent of the iron in vegetable sources, compared with about 15 to 30 percent from meats and fish.

Meats and fish have a second advantage over vegetables. They contain a large percentage of organic *heme* iron, a form of iron the body can absorb intact. Most of the iron in vegetables, grains, and fruit is inorganic *non-heme;* it has to be chemically converted in the stomach and upper part of the small intestine before it's absorbed. Moreover, such foods as eggs, bran, or tea consumed at the same meal will drastically reduce the absorption of non-heme iron. The phytates in cereals and whole wheat bread can also inhibit the body's ability to absorb non-heme iron.

Despite the variety of dietary effects to consider, it's possible to state a few generalizations. A diet that includes only small amounts of meat, poultry, and fish may cause, or at least lead to, iron deficiency. Strict vegetarians and those on a reducing diet that severely restricts caloric intake may not be getting the amount of iron needed. And the consumption of large amounts of "junk foods," which are low in nutrients, may be the cause of both anemia and overweight.

Young women who have started to menstruate are particularly vulnerable. Not only do they lose iron during their menstrual periods, but their iron reserves are additionally strained by the requirements of rapid growth. If they succumb to poor eating habits or go on fad or crash diets, they increase their chances of developing iron deficiency.

Women who find they are in one or more of the "high-risk" categories should not waste their money by dashing out to the nearest drugstore to pick up the first iron supplement they recognize from the ads. Remember, Consumers Union's guidelines are not absolute predictors of iron deficiency. Even an adolescent who menstruates heavily and has a strong preference for candy bars over liver still may be absorbing enough iron to meet her needs. If so, extra iron will not make her healthier; it will be only an unnecessary expense.

The advertised supplements are not the best buys. Late in 1978, CU bought several familiar brands locally and found that such purchases could contribute to a deficiency disease of the pocketbook. For each gram of iron provided, *FemIron* cost $1.99, *Geritol Liquid* cost $2.21, *One a Day Plus Iron* cost $2.58, and *Stresstabs 600 With Iron* cost a stressful $3.08. In contrast, the price for each gram of iron sold in generic form (ferrous sulfate) was only 17 cents. So, buying advertised brands may mean an extra outlay for unneeded vitamins and, in part, paying for more ads.

Accordingly, the generic version, ferrous sulfate, may seem the logical choice for an iron supplement. But even it can present a problem: When used as a supplement, there's simply too much of it. The usual dosage available is equivalent to 60 mg of elemental iron. William Crosby, M.D., an iron expert and chief of hematology at the Scripps Clinic and Research Foundation in La Jolla, California, calls that "an overdose." He says that it makes about 10 percent of its users sick, "either with constipation or diarrhea or upset stomach or dizziness." If the FDA panel has its way, the 60 mg dosage will be earmarked for pregnant women only. *The Medical Letter* suggests supplements of 30 to 60 mg of elemental iron per day (one 300 mg tablet of ferrous sulfate daily or every other day) during the last two trimesters of pregnancy, even for women who are not anemic. For menstruating and lactating women who require iron, the panel-recommended dosage is 10 to 30 mg daily.

Is it simply a question of waiting until the dosage levels of ferrous sulfate tablets come down before you start self-medicating? There's still another catch. The FDA panel recommends the following labeling on OTC iron preparations: "For the prevention of iron deficiency when the need for such therapy has been determined by a physician." Also, the label would include: *"Caution:* The treatment of any anemic condition should be under the advice and supervision of a physician."

As noted earlier, iron-deficiency anemia is hard to self-diagnose. It gives little warning of its approach and few signs of its arrival. But it can be detected, even early on, by a simple, inexpensive blood count that many doctors perform in their office. To detect the anemia before it becomes serious, a blood count every two or three years for all women of childbearing age would be a wise investment of time and money. Routine blood counts are important for women in the "high-risk" categories: Adolescents, heavy menstruaters, and women with diets low in iron.

Women who menstruate heavily may be placed on iron therapy up to menopause. Because of their large monthly iron losses, it may be impossible for them to meet their iron needs without that extra boost. If iron deficiency stems from diet and if eating habits remain unchanged, daily iron therapy may have to become a way of life.

If iron pills are prescribed, keep them in a child-resistant container out of the reach of children. According to the latest figures (1977) from the FDA's Division of Poison Control, at least seventy-five children are hospitalized each year because of accidental iron poisoning. And, according to Crosby, of these seventy-five cases there is a possibility of ten fatalities.

Fortunately, most people don't have to worry about where to store their iron pills. Their iron supply will be in the foods they eat. If dietary iron is too little or iron loss too great, don't look to ads for the answer. If a woman really wants to "take good care" of herself, she will have her physician take a blood count to find out whether treatment is needed.

19

Menstrual tampons and pads

In ancient times, Egyptian women dealt with their menstrual flow by rolling up papyrus leaves and inserting them into the vagina. The Romans used soft wool, while African women used external bandages of grass or vegetable fiber. Some societies simply sent menstruating women to bed, where they lay on toweling; the toweling was burned or buried immediately after use.

By the early 1900s, women were using cloth diapers, which they washed and reused month after month. During World War I, French nurses realized that surgical bandages could be used for absorbing menstrual fluid. After the war, surplus bandage material was packaged as "sanitary" pads. The result was *Kotex,* the first commercially successful disposable product for use during menstruation. *Modess* pads came on the scene a few years later.

A whole new area of competition opened up in the 1930s with the introduction of *Tampax*—an internal tampon with an applicator. Tampons were heralded as a revolutionary advance in hygiene and comfort. They were also denounced as an imminent threat to virginity and morality—a myth that faded with time. New brands of tampons, such as *Playtex* and *Kotex,* were later introduced, and products for internal use steadily gained in popularity. Recently, tampons without applicators, long popular in Europe, began to gain a following here. In March 1978, tampons had a 44 percent share of the menstrual-product market in this country; pads had the rest.

The most recent innovation in menstrual products came in 1970. The conventional pad was reduced in size, stripped of its belt, and equipped with an adhesive band. The result was the mini-pad. Now available in several brands, mini-pads are promoted for use just before menstruation, on days of light flow, and as a supplement to tampons on days of heavy flow. Larger versions known as maxi-pads—conventional-sized pads with the adhesive band for "beltless freedom"—are also marketed. Together, the minis and maxis account for at least half of all pad sales.

There are currently more than 60 tampons and pads available, some of which are sold only in certain areas of the country. (One type of product, the menstrual cup, is no longer manufactured.)

Along with the proliferation in products has come a profusion of advertisements about those products, particularly since a ban on radio and television commercials was lifted in 1972. Some $26 million a year is spent to tout individual brands. Annual expenditures for television commercials have more than doubled since 1975.

The content of magazine ads for menstrual products has changed dramatically in the past few years. Once, a soft-focus photograph of a woman in a long dress, and the words *"Modess,* because . . ." was about as far as advertisers would go. Now, the ads discuss absorbency, insertion, staining, and even "the vaginal opening." Tampons are photographed as they expand in a beaker of water. Cardboard applicators get the same graphic treatment as they unwind.

But there is still a lack of impartial information upon which to base wise buying decisions. Ads aside, the subject of menstrual products is virtually ignored in the media, even in publications aimed at women. This chapter is intended to give women some facts to go on as they decide which product to buy.

An invitation to participate in a Consumers Union survey on tampons and pads was published in *Consumer Reports.* Our information is based on responses received in late 1977 from about 4,500 women—ranging in age from under eighteen to over forty. Each woman filled out a detailed questionnaire about the tampon or pad she was currently using, and about any others she had used within the previous year.

Although our respondents reported on more than sixty products, only twenty-eight were mentioned often enough to form a basis for judgment. The twenty-eight products—fourteen tampons (one of which is no longer available), six conventional pads, three maxi-pads, and five mini-pads—included the most widely sold products in each category.

Our questionnaire covered many aspects of menstrual-product use, but it focused mainly on a number of important attributes of tampons and pads. We asked women to evaluate their product's absorbency, comfort, and ease of use. We also asked whether the product stayed in place, prevented leakage of menstrual fluid, resulted in an unpleasant odor during use, and was visible through clothes.

Finally, we asked the women how easy it was to dispose of the product's wrapper—and applicator, if it had one—and of the product itself after use. (Some products and accessories must be thrown away. Others can be flushed down the toilet if the sewage or septic tank system is in good working order.) Beyond those individual judgments, we asked our respondents to characterize their overall satisfaction with the product.

To supplement our survey findings, we purchased the

twenty-eight products and examined them in the laboratory. We did not, however, perform laboratory tests of absorbency. The usefulness of such measurements is limited. For one thing, they don't take into account individual differences among users. A woman's anatomy, her rate of menstrual flow, the composition of her menstrual fluid, and the way she places the product can drastically affect absorbency. If a woman is very active, a pad or tampon may leak before it has absorbed all the fluid it potentially can.

An additional problem arises with tampons. There are two different methods for testing their absorbency. One involves dunking the tampon into a container of liquid and then weighing the tampon to see how much liquid it retains. The other requires a device called a "Syngyna," which permits testing under simulated vaginal pressure. However, the results of the two tests are frequently at odds with each other. Tampons that expand lengthwise when absorbing fluid (such as *Tampax*) excel in the first. Those that expand in a radial fashion when wet (such as *Playtex* and *Pursettes*) show up well in the second. And neither test does a good job of predicting absorbency in real-life situations.

Our data, on the other hand, do reflect real-life situations. In our analysis of the survey results, we took into account each woman's characterization of her menstrual flow. We based our comparisons on the judgments of women who used a product alone, without "doubling up," on days of heaviest flow. Note, however, that our judgments reflect only the experiences of the women who chose to respond to our survey, and not those of a scientifically selected cross-section of those who use such products.

Some of the answers women gave in the survey led our study in still another direction—to the offices of gynecologists and allergists to check out concerns about the possible health effects of using tampons or pads. Some women were worried that tampons could lead to vaginal or bladder infection, to erosion of the cervix, to hemorrhaging, or to uterine growths. In some cases, their physician had warned them of the supposed danger. But CU's medical consultants rejected all such notions and assured us that neither tampons nor pads are a hazard to health—though tampons should not be used immediately after childbirth and in certain other medical circumstances. In addition, we could find no evidence in the medical literature of health problems occurring during normal use of the products.

Some women are concerned that tampons can somehow "get lost," out of their own and their doctor's reach. But there is no rear exit that tampons can take from the vagina; the passageway through the cervix into the uterus is far too small for a tampon to slip through. A tampon can travel high into a vaginal area beyond the cervix, and its string may disappear from view, but it can always be retrieved by a doctor using a speculum and a long forceps. Some women occasionally forget to remove a tampon and notice a bad odor or discharge a week or so later. But that condition is not serious. Symptoms usually disappear soon after the tampon is removed.

Women have also expressed worry about using "deodorant," or scented, tampons or pads. All of CU's consultants advise against the use of such products because of the possibility of an irritation or allergic reaction. Even women who are not normally sensitive to perfumes may develop a reaction after long use. The genital area is particularly vulnerable because of its moist secretions and lack of circulating air.

Information from the survey supported our consultants' concern. More than 200 respondents had been warned by their doctors not to use deodorant tampons or pads. A number of women reported problems with *Playtex Deodorant Tampons,* the only brand of deodorant tampon in our survey. Of the women who had tried scented *Playtex* in the previous year, 8 percent said they wouldn't use it again because of "medical problems, rash, or infection."

Does the perfume at least provide a benefit for the medical risk involved? Not according to our respondents. They did not rate *Playtex Deodorant Tampons* significantly better in absence of unpleasant odor than the brands without deodorant. In fact, very few women thought using *any* of the tampons resulted in an unpleasant odor. (Since menstrual fluid usually develops an odor only when it's in contact with the air, any unpleasant odor would have to be the result of improper insertion or leakage.)

Of the pads, only two—both mini-pads—were scented. Unpleasant odor was judged less of a problem with *Kotex Deodorant Mini Pads* than with the other brands of mini-pads. The other scented mini-pad, *Carefree Panty Shields,* came out about average on that score. The best way for pad-users to deal with odors, suggest CU's medical consultants, is to use unscented pads and change them frequently.

Apart from some criticism of deodorant products, our respondents were not generally a discontented lot. Most described themselves as "completely satisfied" or "very satisfied" with the product they evaluated. (That positive reaction was not surprising: The women were, by choice, users of those brands at the time they evaluated them and, in most instances, had selected them after trial and error.)

There were levels of satisfaction, however. More women seemed more satisfied with tampons than with conventional pads. Of those who reported using only one type of product, six out of seven preferred tampons. Many of the women who used tampons exclusively gave a number of reasons for their preference. The reasons mentioned most often were comfort, lack of mess and unpleasant odor, invisibility under clothes, ease of use, and ease of disposal. In contrast, most of the women who used pads exclusively gave few reasons—usually just comfort and absorbency. Interestingly, the third most common reason the women gave for preferring pads was "habit"; they said they'd never even tried tampons.

Our survey also revealed differences among the various tampons and pads. Some products scored higher than others on a number of qualities. Others were liked or disliked for one particular reason. And some were mentioned much more frequently than others when we asked which tampons or pads women had tried in the previous year but would *not* want to try again.

Tampons—regular and super. The important difference between regular- and super-sized tampons is really not size, but weight. The supers weigh about 25 percent more than the regulars, which accounts for the greater absorbency of super-sized tampons.

Some tampons have a lubricated tip to help with insertion. Most of the tampons come with a cardboard or plastic applicator, though some have a stick inserter, and some come without any applicator at all. A tampon is designed to be placed a few inches up into the vagina, in its wide, most elastic part. If the tampon is not guided past the constricting muscles at the vaginal opening, it may cause discomfort. Once it's past those muscles, a slight tug on the string will "set" it against the muscles, minimizing any leakage.

Of the tampons without applicators, *O.B.* and *Pursettes* did well on our question dealing with disposability. *Playtex* tampons did poorly on that question; some users were apparently unhappy that they couldn't simply flush the product's plastic applicator down the toilet and be done with it.

O.B. users commented negatively on "ease of use." It is

possible that these women, lured by *O.B.* advertising, were unaccustomed to a tampon without an applicator. Regular-sized *Pursettes,* which also come without an applicator, had a wide range of reactions: Although more than 80 percent of the product's current users described themselves as completely satisfied or very satisfied, half of the women who had used the product in the previous year said they wouldn't try it again, usually because it was "difficult to insert." For any of the other products, the dropout figure did not exceed 31 percent.

Pads—regular and super. Pads are held in place by an elastic belt worn over the hips. Clasps hold the pad in front and in back. The pads we looked at had a plastic shield to help keep the fluid from leaking out. The three brands varied somewhat in shape: *Kotex* and *Modess,* basically rectangular; *Confidets,* with a tapering-V shape.

As with tampons, super-sized pads achieve increased absorbency by increased weight. The difference is most dramatic for *Modess:* The super-sized pads are almost 30 percent heavier than the regulars.

In the regular size category, *Confidets Sanitary Napkins* came out way ahead of both *Modess Feminine Napkins* and *Kotex Feminine Napkins,* excelling in practically all the qualities we asked about. Super-sized *Confidets* were also preferred, but to a lesser extent. *Modess* was in second place in both size categories, scoring higher than *Kotex* in overall satisfaction and in many specific attributes. Interestingly, the order of satisfaction reversed that of sales. *Kotex* is by far the biggest seller of the three; *Confidets,* the smallest.

Confidets pads and wrappers were judged much easier to dispose of than the other brands. *Confidets* comes with individual disposal bags, apparently an appealing feature to many of the product's users. None of the conventional pads, maxi-pads, or mini-pads can be flushed away; their bulk and their plastic shield prevent that.

When we asked which products a woman had tried in the previous year and would not want to try again, we found that a much higher percentage of women had been dissatisfied with *Kotex* than with either *Confidets* or *Modess*. (Since our survey, *Kotex* has come out with "improved" pads. In CU's judgment, however, the differences between old and new *Kotex* pads appear very slight.)

Maxi-pads. These products are similar to conventional pads in size, and they weigh just slightly less than the regular-sized versions. Instead of a belt, they have one or more adhesive strips that attach to underwear. Like the belted pads, they have a plastic shield to guard against leakage.

None of the three maxi-pads mentioned most often by our respondents was much preferred over the others. *Kotex Maxi Pads* scored significantly better than *New Freedom Maxi Pads* on just one factor—ability to protect against leakage. Yet both products are essentially the same shape, size, and weight. And *Kotex* was judged more comfortable than *Stayfree Maxi-Pads*. (The two products are shaped somewhat differently; *Kotex* is less rounded at the ends than *Stayfree* and tapers off in thickness at front and back.) Nevertheless, one out of five women who used *Kotex* in the previous year said they wouldn't try it again—a slightly higher proportion than for *New Freedom* or *Stayfree*.

Mini-pads. This innovation apparently has met with very wide acceptance. Eight out of ten women surveyed had used the small, lightweight pads at one time or another, and more than three-quarters of those women still were using them.

Most women said they wore mini-pads chiefly on days of light menstrual flow. A smaller group wore them just before menstruation, or for extra protection on days of heavy flow. In evaluating our survey results, we focused on their main use: For days of light menstrual flow.

As with the maxi-pads, no one brand was higher in overall satisfaction. *Carefree Panty Shields,* which is one-eighth inch thick (most of the other minis are one-half inch thick), scored a little higher on several of the qualities we asked about. *Kotex Light Days,* which is only one-sixteenth inch thick, was judged below average in absorbency, comfort, and absence of unpleasant odor.

Most of the women responding to our survey strongly preferred tampons. To women who have never used tampons, our first recommendation is to give them a try. Among tampons, regular and super *Carefree* were much preferred over other brands. The product is no longer available, but its replacement, *O.B.,* is identical to it in shape and size. *O.B.* fared less well with our respondents, but that may be because it was, in 1977, a new product that women were not yet used to. Both *Carefree* and *O.B.* come without an applicator. No brand of tampon with an applicator was preferred over any other; most were judged average in the various qualities we asked about.

For women who like using conventional pads: Consider switching to regular or super *Confidets,* which many of our respondents preferred to *Modess* or *Kotex.* Among maxi- and mini-pads, there were essentially no differences in overall satisfaction.

A local survey by CU shoppers indicated that price differences are generally small for pads—not more than a penny or two a pad separates brands. The price range is slightly larger among brands of tampons, with deodorant versions by far the most expensive. And CU's medical consultants believe that you can save in more ways than one by avoiding deodorized menstrual products.

20
Genital deodorants for women

In the 1960s the cosmetic industry realized that its valiant—and profitable—campaign to ban body odor could be extended beyond the underarm area. By 1966 the genital deodorant was ready for its commercial debut; soon corner drugstores were displaying rows of genital deodorant sprays for women (and even brands for men). The age of the genital cosmetic flowered, and by 1971 there were thirty brands of "feminine hygiene spray" (the euphemism for women's genital deodorants) for which Americans were willing to spend $67.7 million.

A typical feminine deodorant spray at one time included an emollient acting as a carrier, a propellant, and a perfume. No one could be positive about the ingredients because under the then existing law a "cosmetic" product did not need to list all —or any—of its ingredients on the label. After April 15, 1977, however, the Food and Drug Administration (FDA) enforced a requirement that labels for newly manufactured cosmetics include information about ingredients. Until September 1972, when the FDA banned use of hexachlorophene in over-the-counter products, many formulations included hexachlorophene. However, most manufacturers of genital sprays never replaced the banned chemical with other antibacterial agents.

Even today, when consumers are no longer frightened of genital odor and more informed about the hazards of the product, sales figures indicate the business is still somewhat profitable. In 1975 the total spent on genital deodorants was $20.3 million; by 1976 the figure had been reduced to $17.2 million; and by the end of 1977 the figure had dropped to a mere $14.7 million—perhaps reflecting the record of painful injuries, discomfort, and irritations attributed to use of the product and indicating its diminishing availability in the marketplace.

Another probable factor in the sales dip was the influence of women who resisted the sales pitch. For example, Germaine Greer, author of *The Female Eunuch,* dismissed the deodorants with the comment that she had never seen anyone lying around overcome by vaginal fumes. Other leaders of the women's movement joined in condemning the vaginal spray as a totally useless and demeaning product. Natalie Shainess, M.D., a New York psychiatrist, said at a Senate hearing in 1971, "While fostering an overt message of a feminine, 'sexy' woman, the implication of need for such a spray conveys a message of woman as being dirty and smelly—extremely damaging to a woman's sense of self."

The initial sales success of genital deodorants can be attributed to more than the American preoccupation with how people smell or the increasingly relaxed attitudes towards sex. Madison Avenue's ability to create a market also played a part. The uninhibited advertising for genital cosmetics reflected the ingenuity of copywriters in selling the wares of their new clients. According to many of the advertisements, not only did genital sprays enhance a woman's sex appeal, but they also kept her from being downright offensive.

The advertising copy in vogue several years ago was downright demeaning. Warner-Lambert's *Pristeen* genital spray warned, "Unfortunately, the trickiest deodorant problem a girl has *isn't* under her pretty little arms." The personal products division of Johnson & Johnson advertised its female genital spray, *Vespré*, as "the intimate odor preventive." ("Some sprays hide it. Some sprays mask it, but *Vespré* actually prevents intimate odor.") Regardless of what it could or could not do, *Vespré* is no longer around: Johnson & Johnson took it off the market.

Television advertising for genital deodorants alone reached an annual rate of $10 million by 1971. In typical Madison Avenue style, the demand had actually been created for a new product. "In this world of accelerating change, new ideas and new products are constantly originated that contribute to the betterment of our lives and broadening of our horizons," reported the president of Alberto-Culver, manufacturer of *FDS* (a leading product in the field).

Bernard A. Davis, M.D., a Montreal gynecologist, was less enthusiastic about this latest contribution to the full life. He reported treating about thirty cases of inflammation of the genital area following the use of feminine sprays. "Surely," he said, "in this gadget-conscious, product-oriented civilization, we must resist those instances where a demand is being artificially created for a product of questionable value. This is especially true where even the minimal advantage can be more than outweighed by significant complications."

The president of Alberto-Culver said, in defense of female genital deodorants, that they solved a problem dating from biblical times. The "problem," as seen from the manufacturer's vantage point, was as old as woman herself. The external genitals, the vulva, contain glands capable of producing mildly odorous secretions. Close-fitting underwear, pantyhose, or tight slacks tend to delay evaporation of perspiration. Normal skin bacteria act on those secretions and produce an odor that the cosmetic industry would have women regard as unpleasant.

Most healthy women have natural vulval odors to greater or lesser degree. Consumers Union's medical consultants advise soap and water as the most effective and certainly the safest hygiene for vulval odors that occur naturally. And *The Medical Letter* states, "It is unlikely that commercial feminine hygiene sprays are as effective as soap and water in promoting a hygienic and odor-free external genital surface."

Usually vaginal infections give rise to foul-smelling discharges. Less commonly, an unsuspected tumor of the uterus or cervix may produce secretions that are also malodorous. Some odors may be due to the presence of a foreign body, such as a forgotten tampon or diaphragm. Occasionally menstrual flow itself may be accompanied by malodor. Soap and water may not take care of odors from these causes. But neither will a chemical spray. Indeed, the use of a genital deodorant may discourage some people from washing often enough. And most important, CU's medical consultants are concerned that the use of genital sprays may make some women with medically significant odorous vaginal discharges put off seeking medical advice while using the sprays instead.

Advertising has at times hinted that genital deodorants should be sprayed directly into the vagina instead of onto the *external* genital area. Such internal use could be especially dangerous. According to Bernard M. Kaye, M.D., a gynecologist formerly with the Abraham Lincoln School of Medicine of the University of Illinois, "There is an implication of vaginal use in the names of the products and the advertising. Vaginal use is absolutely contraindicated and will lead to irritation from the propellant and/or the ingredients of the product."

Again as a result of advertising, women may believe that the moment prior to sexual intercourse is the ideal time to make use of this "cosmetic" product. CU's medical consultants warn that it is particularly ill-advised to apply a female genital deodorant just before intercourse because there is the chance that the freshly sprayed chemicals might be carried into the vagina. Moreover, according to *Today's Health,* an American Medical Association publication, there have been reports of male genital irritation attributable to intercourse with a partner who had used a genital spray deodorant immediately before.

In a letter to *The New England Journal of Medicine* in July 1972, John M. Gowdy, M.D., formerly of the FDA's food division, which has jurisdiction over cosmetics, reported that a variety of complaints about genital deodorant sprays had been received by his agency, and noted, "The offending ingredient has not been identified." Gowdy stated that, although the reactions were not life-threatening, "all were locally severe, and average recovery time was thirty days." Gowdy added that pressure from propellants "may be important" in setting up local inflammation of the urethra (the short passage leading from the bladder).

Such inflammations may result in narrowing of the urethra, which not only can cause painful urination but, more important, can lead to consequent retention of urine within the bladder. This in turn leads to recurrent urinary tract infections, which, as many women know, can be troublesome and difficult to cure with medication, and may sometimes require dilatation of the urethra or other surgical treatment.

In January 1972, *Consumer Reports* published an article on genital deodorants, describing them as potentially hazardous and documenting its case with reports of injuries and serious harm. (Because these products had been classified as "cosmetics," rather than drugs, they escaped the extensive premarketing test programs required of all new drugs to establish their safety and effectiveness.) It was some time before the FDA took any action. Finally, in June 1973, more than a year after CU first broke the story on the dangers in using genital sprays, the FDA proposed that a mandatory warning be required on every package. The FDA also took note of the misleading "hygiene" or "hygienic" terminology usually tacked onto the descriptions of these products, and denied manufacturers the right to use such terminology with its implication of medical benefit. However, the FDA did not reclassify genital sprays as drugs but permitted them to remain in the cosmetic category and thus to continue to be sold to consumers many of whom might not read the warnings on the label. (The FDA stated that products manufactured after November 30, 1976, were to carry new labels.)

Most authorities would go further than the mandatory warning the FDA required for these products. Even the FDA's own advisory panel of obstetricians and gynecologists voted unanimously in October 1972 that genital deodorants should be considered drugs and therefore made subject to extensive controlled testing for safety and effectiveness before further marketing would be permitted. The FDA warning, intended "to minimize any possible risk to users," does take one very minimal step to deal with possible hazards to users. It included a recommendation that the spray be kept at least 8 inches from the skin instead of the 6 inches recommended on labels prior to the new requirements.

Although many people may be able to use genital deodorants without apparent ill effect, there is always a risk involved in applying chemicals to the surface of the skin, especially to such sensitive areas as the external genitals. But manufacturers of genital deodorants tended to shrug off any possible risk as insignificant. Warner-Lambert, the makers of *Pristeen,* and Alberto-Culver said they received adverse reactions at a rate of only six per million sales. Even at that rate, as of April 1971 Alberto-Culver had reports of 107 women users of *FDS* who had complained of irritation, allergic reactions, burns, infection, dermatitis of the thighs, stinging, swelling, itching, inflammation, lumps, and even a burned hand. (Alberto-Culver had to furnish this information to a court in connection with a lawsuit filed by a woman who claimed to have been injured by *FDS*.)

The number of complaints probably understated the problem. Most people, after all, did not bother to write; they merely stopped using the product. A few might have consulted a doctor, never suspecting that the deodorant was the real cause of their discomfort. Kaye reported in the periodical *Medical Aspects of Human Sexuality* on interviews with twenty patients: Fourteen said they had used a genital spray deodorant; of the fourteen, four reported vulval itching or burning.

Some reported cases went beyond mere discomfort. One fourteen-year-old girl was described by her physician as having suffered "incredibly" from swollen labia. In one of at least two lawsuits filed against Alberto-Culver, a woman who used *FDS* spray alleged that she quickly developed large lumps and had to be admitted to a hospital when the condition became so painful that she had difficulty walking. Her doctor diagnosed the problem as a severe reaction to *FDS* spray. "The swelling was as big as a grapefruit," her physician said. "You never saw a more miserable girl in your life." Her lawsuit against Alberto-Culver was settled out of court.

When a college student wrote to Alberto-Culver asking about the risk of adverse reactions to *FDS* spray, the company told her, "While the occurrence of such reactions is rare compared to the number of people who use the products regularly, they do occasionally occur and can be quite painful." The firm called attention to its label directions instructing the user to hold the can about 6 inches from the body while spraying. Then it added some information not found on the label: "Holding the spray too close might deposit a concentrated amount of the spray on the body and this could cause some irritation."

In view of such possibilities, what kind of safety testing was done before the genital deodorant was brought to the market?

An indication of the type of testing necessary was supplied in a technical article by John A. Cella, Ph.D., who was then Alberto-Culver vice-president for consumer product research, in the October 1971 issue of *American Perfumer and Cosmetics*. "In formulating deodorant products, as with all toiletries, sufficient testing should be done *in vitro* [sic] in animals and humans to assure that the product is safe for repeated use and is effective in delivering the label claims," he wrote. According to Cella, "minimum testing" for a female genital spray "should include animal skin irritation and sensitization studies, animal vulvar irritation studies, animal vaginal instillation studies using the aerosol concentrates, human repeated insult patch tests on intact and abraded skin, subacute and chronic human use tests, particle size analysis of the spray and animal inhalation studies." Cella also called for extensive laboratory and use tests to determine the effectiveness of female genital sprays.

Despite Cella's call for extensive safety testing, Alberto-Culver's sworn pretrial statement in the aforementioned lawsuit did *not* include most of his test proposals when it outlined the testing done prior to the marketing of *FDS* in 1966. Furthermore, an FDA medical officer who reviewed the Alberto-Culver data disagreed sharply with the company's conclusions and stated: "Thus while close to 25 percent of the subjects seemed to have some type of adverse reaction to the product, the company reports no irritation or other abnormality."

In 1971 in response to a questionnaire from CU, Alberto-Culver listed several tests it claimed to have conducted *after* introducing *FDS* on the market. However, they hardly compensated for the totally inadequate premarket test program set forth in the pretrial testimony. Had the FDA agreed to reclassify female genital sprays as drugs—instead of merely requiring that a warning label be affixed—manufacturers would have been required to provide evidence concerning the safety and effectiveness of their products. The nature of that evidence might have proved embarrassing for the entire deodorant industry if Alberto-Culver's premarket test program had been at all typical.

Problems of safety in using genital deodorants are part of the larger picture of cosmetics and their hazards. The best solution to these problems is stronger cosmetics legislation.

In June 1975 the FDA set regulations for the marketing of cosmetics labeled as "hypoallergenic." After June 6, 1977, all manufacturers were to be required to submit evidence of clinical testing to substantiate claims that their products cause fewer adverse reactions in human subjects than competing brands. The two makers of "hypoallergenic" cosmetics (Almay and Clinique) filed suit in U.S. District Court for the District of Columbia in July 1975. The court upheld the FDA regulations, but the two companies appealed. In its December 1977 decision, the appeals court reversed the district court ruling, maintaining that the FDA's definition of the term "hypoallergenic" was unreasonable because the FDA had not demonstrated that consumers perceive the term in the way described in the regulations. The FDA plans no further action on these proposed regulations.

Meanwhile, the FDA proposed a solution as of May 30, 1975, that called for a two-part schedule to implement ingredient labeling of all cosmetic products. Part 1 called for all labels ordered by cosmetic manufacturers after May 31, 1976, to have a listing of ingredients. Part 2 required all new cosmetics to which labels are affixed after November 30, 1976, to have a listing of ingredients. Part 1 went into effect as scheduled. Part

2, however, was held up by a challenge from the Independent Cosmetic Manufacturers and Distributors that resulted in court action. The challenge was defeated and Part 2 went into effect April 15, 1977. People with allergies and those hypersensitive to certain chemicals would be wise to check the labels on all cosmetics before buying them.

The one cosmetic consumers can surely do without—even with its ingredients clearly marked on the label—is the genital deodorant.

21
Pregnancy test kits

There was a time when a woman who wondered if she were pregnant either waited for obvious physical signs or consulted a physician. Now she can walk into a drugstore and buy a do-it-yourself kit. The kit, called *EPT* for "early pregnancy test," is marketed by Warner/Chilcott, a division of the Warner-Lambert Co. The *EPT* kit, a urine test, can be used only once. In November 1978, it cost from $9.95 to $10.95; in June 1979, the price range was $7.19 to $10.95.

Warner/Chilcott has promoted the *EPT* with full-page advertisements in magazines addressed to women, trumpeting it as "a private little revolution any woman can easily buy at her drugstore." But is the revolution really at hand? It's doubtful —for a variety of reasons.

Until about fifty years ago pregnancy detection relied on the classic signs of early pregnancy: Missed menstrual period, morning sickness, breast tenderness, and others. In the 1920s, a test was developed in which a woman's urine was injected into laboratory animals (eventually it became known as the "rabbit test"). A pregnant woman's urine contains a hormone —human chorionic gonadotropin, or HCG—that causes observable changes in the animal's reproductive organs.

In 1960, scientists developed a laboratory test—a pregnancy "immunoassay"—which can be performed in a test tube or on a slide. In a test-tube immunoassay, a few drops of a woman's urine are added to a test tube containing antibodies against HCG. If HCG is present in the urine, it combines with the antibodies, causing a brown ring to form at the bottom of the test tube. This is a "positive" result, indicating pregnancy. The immunoassay has become the most widely used pregnancy test, because it is faster, less expensive, and more convenient than animal tests.

The *EPT* is simply a test-tube immunoassay. It's "revolutionary" only in that it was the first immunoassay available in this country for use in the home rather than in a laboratory or a doctor's office. Nearly identical do-it-yourself pregnancy test kits have been sold in Europe and Canada since the early 1970s. In fact, the *EPT* is actually manufactured by a Dutch company; Warner/Chilcott imports the kits, repackages them, and sells them under its own name.

In 1976 Congress gave the Food and Drug Administration (FDA) authority to rule on the safety and effectiveness of all medical devices. According to an FDA official, the *EPT* was rushed onto the market a few days before the Medical Device Amendments of 1976 became operative. Since the law was not retroactive, *EPT* could continue to be marketed without FDA approval.

What information can a do-it-yourself test give? A sexually active woman with regular menstrual cycles knows that a delay in the onset of menstruation may mean she is pregnant. The *EPT* and similar tests could help resolve the issue—provided the test results were reliable. Warner/Chilcott's studies carried out on the *EPT* indicate that 97 percent of the women who get a positive result actually were pregnant. Thus the test can be accurate when it is positive.

But what about a negative test result? According to a study described in the *EPT* instruction pamphlet, a negative result offers no assurance that a woman is *not* pregnant. The study showed that 20 percent of the women who got negative *EPT* results were in fact pregnant. The percentage of "false negatives" was even higher, 25 percent, in a second study conducted by Warner/Chilcott but not included in the pamphlet. That high an incidence of false negatives makes the *EPT* unreliable, in the view of Consumers Union's medical consultants.

One reason for the high incidence of false negatives, CU suspects, is the instructions given in the pamphlet that comes with the kit. The pamphlet urges a woman to use the kit as early as the ninth day after her menstrual period should have begun. The HCG hormone is undetectable at the start of pregnancy but steadily increases in the blood and urine until it reaches its maximum level at about ten weeks after conception. So the earlier a pregnant woman uses the kit, the more likely she is to get a false negative result. And the chance of her getting a false negative result on the earliest day—day nine —is much greater than the 20 to 25 percent chance reported by Warner/Chilcott.

From a sales perspective, the *EPT* pitch of "the earlier you know, the better," is understandable. Some pregnant women will use a kit before the HCG hormone is detectable in their urine. Then, if they follow the package insert's advice about what to do if the test is negative, they will buy a second kit and repeat the test a week later. However, a woman's menstruation can be delayed for various reasons other than pregnancy, such as illness, emotional upset, or weight loss. And as many as half of all women whose period is nine days late end up menstruating. Therefore, many nonpregnant women may needlessly buy and use one or more of the kits.

Ads for the *EPT* claim that women will benefit from "early knowledge of pregnancy." One ad says that the kit can help women "control the quality of their pregnancies." It correctly points out that cigarettes, alcohol, and commonly used medications might harm the fetus during the crucial first weeks of pregnancy and that early knowledge of pregnancy could help women avoid these substances. However, immunoassays such as the *EPT* usually cannot detect pregnancy until a woman has been pregnant for about three to four weeks. Knowledge at that time would certainly be helpful, but users should know that by then some harmful substances might already have damaged developing fetal organs. Would early knowledge of pregnancy result in better prenatal care? According to CU's medical consultants, routine obstetrical care can usually wait until four to six weeks after the first missed period.

What about women who fear an unwanted pregnancy? If they use the *EPT* as early as the manufacturer recommends, they risk getting a false negative result—and false reassurance. Yet, there's really no medical reason to find out so soon. Recent studies show that the risk of complications from an abortion is lowest when it is performed about four weeks after the first missed period.

For these reasons, we recommend that if a woman chooses to use such a kit at all, she should wait until her period is fourteen days late if her cycle is regular and twenty-one days late if her cycle is irregular. The extra few days' wait makes it more likely that the urinary HCG level will be high enough to be detected by the test. That will reduce the chance of a false negative result—and the need to perform a second test.

If a woman is not pregnant, waiting the extra days may save her the expense of a pregnancy test. Her period may well occur during this time—and that's usually the most reliable indicator that she is not pregnant. (In a small percentage of women, some menstrual bleeding may occur early in pregnancy.)

To use the *EPT,* a woman must follow a nine-step procedure that allows ample opportunity for error. For example, the test tube and its contents must stand perfectly still for exactly two hours before the result can be "read" in the bottom of the tube. According to the instructions, the test can give an inaccurate result if the slightest vibration occurs or if the result is read too early or too late.

Even if it is used correctly, the *EPT* appears to be a needless purchase. A positive result on either the first or second try indicates pregnancy, and pregnancy indicates that a visit to a physician is in order. CU spoke with several obstetricians. All would insist, they said, on confirming the diagnosis with another pregnancy test. So the woman with a positive *EPT* result ends up paying for an obstetrician's pregnancy test anyway. If she had telephoned the doctor in the first place or used any of the low-cost methods described later in this chapter, she probably would have paid for only one pregnancy test.

A negative *EPT* result is even less useful. That merely tells a woman she *might* not be pregnant; she certainly must still await menstruation or other confirmation.

There is a test that's better than the urinary immunoassay method for early diagnosis of pregnancy. It's called the radioreceptor assay. Unlike the conventional test, the radioreceptor assay requires a blood sample and is nearly 100 percent accurate at about the time of the first missed period. It can even detect pregnancy a few days before the period is due. The test usually costs from $10 to $15. Because it requires expensive laboratory equipment, it's generally available only in medical centers and in large commercial laboratories. The test may be especially useful for women who need to know their pregnancy status as early as possible, such as those scheduled to undergo X rays, drug therapy, or surgery.

Women who favor do-it-yourself pregnancy tests such as the *EPT* may believe that professional testing is inconvenient and expensive. A survey conducted for Diagnostic Testing Co., which markets *Answer,* a pregnancy test kit, found that most of those interested in the kits were middle-income married women in their early thirties. According to a Diagnostic Testing representative, these women gave roughly the following argument for buying an OTC pregnancy test kit.

> If I think I'm pregnant, I have to call my doctor, and then I'm lucky to get an appointment within two weeks. When I go to the doctor's office I have to take off a half-day or a full day from work, which comes out of my sick leave. Then, after sitting in the waiting room for an hour and a half, I finally get in to see the doctor. The doctor orders a pregnancy test done on me, and I can only find out the result by calling back two days later. In two weeks, I get a doctor's bill of from $25 to $40 for an office visit and a separate lab bill for $15.

Is that an accurate view of the health-care system for a woman who wants a pregnancy test? Not necessarily. A CU staffer telephoned the offices of fourteen obstetricians in suburban New York and Connecticut in the fall of 1978 and told each she wanted to find out if she were pregnant. Three of them said she could drop off a urine specimen at their office any morning and call back that afternoon to learn the result. No appointment was needed and the cost was $8 to $10— about the cost of the *EPT.* One of the three had a "drop box" outside the door so that a woman didn't even have to walk into the office. The other eleven doctors referred our reporter to a nearby hospital or laboratory—nine for a blood test (the very accurate radioreceptor assay mentioned earlier) and two for a urine test. Cost: $10 to $15. And the results could be had by phone the same day for samples obtained that morning.

As our telephone calls suggest, a woman doesn't need to have a personal physician in order to obtain a test through a doctor. Moreover, there are many other places to go for a professional, confidential, and inexpensive pregnancy test.

The Planned Parenthood Federation of America, Inc., has more than 700 centers across the country offering pregnancy testing and other services. Some centers charge a fixed fee, while others have a sliding scale depending on the patient's income. All centers offer free testing to those who cannot afford it. Typical cost was $5 to $10 in June 1979, and patients could get the result before they left. Planned Parenthood also offers free counseling to anyone having questions about pregnancy, family planning, fertility problems, and other related topics. Some of the affiliates offer a free second pregnancy test as well if the first one is negative. To assure an accurate diagnosis, Planned Parenthood also urges its patients to have a pelvic examination within ten days after the test.

Many state, county, and city health departments offer inexpensive and confidential pregnancy testing, usually as part of their family planning programs. In Maryland, for example, each county health department offers pregnancy testing. Patients who can't afford the test pay nothing, and in most counties in late 1978 the maximum charge for others was $6 to $8. Patients are also entitled to additional pregnancy tests at no extra cost, and to free counseling and referral for follow-up services. According to one state health official: "There is no reason for a woman in Maryland to buy a kit such as the *EPT* unless she doesn't want to be seen at the health department."

Many hospitals and neighborhood health centers offer professional pregnancy testing at prices lower than the price of the *EPT,* although a doctor's referral is often necessary. If you are not sure where such testing is offered in your community, ask the local health department or county medical society.

22
Drugs
in pregnancy

Prior to 1962 generations of physicians were taught the comforting myth that the placenta—the organ within the uterus through which a fetus receives its nourishment—was a sort of guardian angel, a St. Peter at the gates of the umbilical cord, passing needed nutrients through while holding back harmful germs and chemicals. It was long known, of course, that there were some exceptions. Rubella (German measles) virus, for instance, could be transmitted from a pregnant woman to an embryo in the first three months (trimester) of pregnancy, causing defects in the fetus. But not until 1962 did many physicians pay serious attention to the possibility that other dangerous substances might be passed from pregnant women to fetus.

In that year the world was shocked to learn that thalidomide, a drug then commonly prescribed in many countries for insomnia and nervous tension, was in fact a teratogen—a substance capable of producing malformations in a fetus. Babies born to women who took thalidomide early in pregnancy suffered from phocomelia, or "seal limbs"—so called because foreshortened arms and legs resembling the flippers of seals are the most conspicuous result.

Rather than being a barrier to the transfer of drugs from pregnant woman to fetus, "the placenta is a sieve," said the late Virginia Apgar, M.D., then vice-president for medical research of The National Foundation–March of Dimes. Apgar added, "Almost everything ingested by or injected into the mother can be expected to reach the fetus within a few minutes." Alcohol, antibiotics, aspirin, barbiturates, sulfonamides, and tranquilizers are but a few of the common, and possibly harmful, substances known to pass through the placenta. Moreover, certain drugs can be found in even greater concentration in the fetal brain, heart muscle, or other organs than in the maternal tissues. In addition, the capacity of the placenta to allow transfer of some drugs seems to increase with the duration of pregnancy.

Much of this information had long been known to the relatively small group of investigators who studied the physiology of the human fetus; but little of their knowledge filtered through to practicing physicians, or even to those responsible for setting the requirements of drug testing. It took the thalidomide disaster to secure wide clinical acceptance of the established facts of fetal physiology. Physicians today assume that, when they prescribe a drug for a pregnant woman, the drug or its breakdown products—with few known exceptions—will also circulate through the fetus.

When pictures of thalidomide babies first hit the front pages of newspapers, many pregnant women were dismayed and immediately discontinued whatever medication they had been taking. It may be that some pregnant women still refuse to take any drugs at all.

Consumers Union's medical consultants agree that those who are pregnant—and those who wish to become pregnant—should avoid virtually all medication *for the relief of minor symptoms,* especially during the first trimester of pregnancy.

However, those who are in need of medical treatment or already under the care of a doctor should be guided by their physician. Pregnant women can have any disease other women have. Tuberculosis, diabetes, infectious diseases such as syphilis and gonorrhea, heart disease, epilepsy—these are but a few of the diseases that, if left untreated during pregnancy, may affect a fetus. Thus CU's medical consultants stress the importance both of taking prescribed medicines and of refraining from unnecessary medication.

A diabetic is a prime example of the type of patient who needs close medical supervision during pregnancy. CU's medical consultants suggest that diabetics make arrangements for medical care as early as possible in their pregnancy. Those with milder forms of the disease may do perfectly well on a special diet and without specific medication. Those patients who are on insulin and become pregnant usually continue to take this injectable drug, which is considered safe for use in pregnancy. Those who have been taking oral diabetes medication, however, may have to switch to insulin for the duration of their pregnancy. The safety during pregnancy of such oral medications as tolbutamide (Orinase) and acetohexamide (Dymelor) has not been established. Indeed, the long-term safety of these drugs for the general diabetic population has come under serious question by some researchers as well as the Food and Drug Administration (FDA).

"Why don't they test new drugs first on pregnant laboratory animals before permitting their use by pregnant women?" This question was often asked at the height of the thalidomide tragedy, and one of the results of the tragedy has been improvements in animal test procedures.

The FDA guidelines for the evaluation of new drugs for use in pregnancy, announced in 1966, were stricter and better designed than earlier FDA recommendations. The guidelines even specified that a new drug be administered to male animals to check its effect on their sperm cells and their offspring. But as more and more animal tests have been run, it has become increasingly apparent that the results of tests on animals may not always apply to humans.

That does not mean that animal tests are worthless for human protection. They can serve to arouse suspicion and to remind physicians of the need for caution. But no drug can be considered safe during pregnancy unless it has actually been administered to pregnant women under carefully controlled conditions, and until the babies born to these women have been carefully studied for a period of years to check for defects not diagnosable at birth or during infancy.

Since controlled experiments on pregnant women are quite properly frowned upon, the degree of hazard associated with the vast array of drugs in current use has never been adequately investigated. This is why the precautions suggested by CU's medical consultants are phrased in terms of all drugs rather than selected groups of drugs.

Some drugs, such as diethylstilbestrol (DES)—see page 254 —prevent implantation of the fertilized ovum in the wall of the uterus, if used in sufficiently high dosage. They thus act as postcoital contraceptives if their use is begun within seventy-two hours after sexual intercourse. But the possibility exists that a woman who *wants* to become pregnant may use a drug that could also have this contraceptive effect, or other as yet undiscovered effects, during the period immediately following conception.

Accordingly, CU's medical consultants recommend that a fertile woman who is sexually active think of herself as potentially pregnant if she does not use contraceptive measures— and if she would not wish to abort the pregnancy should conception occur. She should discuss with her physician any drug that may be prescribed, and at the same time restrict her use of nonprescription drugs. In this way she would enhance the likelihood of having a healthy baby, should she become pregnant.

Most fetal malformations, of course, are caused by factors other than drugs and are not easily avoided. But drug-caused malformations *are* avoidable. The thalidomide disaster served to focus popular attention on one kind of drug-related malformation—the kind likely to follow when a drug is taken between the third and twelfth weeks of pregnancy. During these crucial weeks the fetus begins to assume recognizable form; the basic structures of the brain, heart, arms, legs, eyes, glands, and other organs are laid down day by day. As a result, the malformations produced also vary, depending on the stage of fetal development at which the pregnant woman took the drug.

The FDA has warned doctors that certain minor tranquilizers—meprobamate (Equanil, Miltown), chlordiazepoxide (Librium), and diazepam (Valium)—should not be prescribed for pregnant patients. Valium is the most commonly prescribed drug in the United States, and Librium is close behind. According to the FDA, 6.5 million prescriptions a month are written for these two drugs alone. (Studies have shown that 60 to 70 percent of all tranquilizer prescriptions are written for women.) The FDA has ordered the manufacturers of these drugs to include a label warning against their prescription during the first three months of pregnancy. Recent studies have suggested that there might be an association between use of these drugs and fetal malformations, such as cleft lip. Because of the increased incidence of birth defects found in babies born to mothers for whom these minor tranquilizers have been prescribed, women who wish to become pregnant should inform their doctors so that suspect drugs are not prescribed during early fetal development.

Examples of other drugs that may be hazardous in the early stages of pregnancy are antinausea medications, such as meclizine (Bonine) and cyclizine (Marezine). These drugs can cause fetal abnormalities in experimental animals. Although there is no evidence of harm to human beings, CU's medical consultants advise against their use by pregnant or potentially pregnant women.

Other well-known medications, including anticonvulsants such as diphenylhydantoin (Dilantin), have been found to be associated with an increased frequency of congenital malformations.

All women, especially pregnant women, should be wary of metronidazole (Flagyl), a drug for treatment of a vaginal infection and sold as pills and as vaginal inserts. Studies have shown it to be carcinogenic in laboratory animals; other studies suggest possible genetic damage. Methotrexate, a potent medication that has been prescribed for certain types of cancer, has been used to treat severe cases of psoriasis. Women for whom methotrexate has been prescribed should be aware that instances of fetal malformation due to this medication have been well documented. Other anticancer drugs, including azathioprine (Imuran), cyclophosphamide (Cytoxan), and mercaptopurine (Purinethol), when taken in the first few months of pregnancy, have been associated with a high rate of miscarriage.

Vaccination against rubella is contraindicated for pregnant women. Administration of rubella vaccine in the early stages of pregnancy carries a theoretical risk of fetal abnormalities. CU's medical consultants advise women who are vaccinated against rubella to avoid becoming pregnant for three months following vaccination. Women who expect to become pregnant and who are concerned about whether they need vaccination against rubella should be tested for the presence of antibodies if there is no adequate proof of having had rubella in childhood. A sample of blood can be submitted to a laboratory; many state laboratories perform the test without cost. If the test detects the presence of rubella antibodies, the vaccine need not be administered. The Center for Disease Control (CDC) in Atlanta reports that the following states require blood tests of women who are planning to marry, in order to determine their susceptibility to rubella: California, Colorado, Connecticut, Georgia, Hawaii, Idaho, Maine, Massachusetts, and Rhode Island. (North Carolina repealed its law in 1979.)

Because rubella and thalidomide—the two most publicized causes of prenatal malformations—have been identified as hazards in the first trimester of pregnancy, many people have gained the impression that drugs taken during other stages of pregnancy are harmless. Not so. While malformations arise mostly during the first three months of pregnancy—even before the first menstrual period is missed—hazards of other kinds can occur during the later stages of pregnancy.

One authority has characterized the second trimester as "the great unknown." However, two examples of drug-induced damage during the second trimester can be cited. Certain hormones of the class known as progestational agents, formerly prescribed in an attempt to avert miscarriage, sometimes produce masculinizing effects such as enlargement of the clitoris in the female fetus. (Such variations can be surgically corrected.) Substances such as iodides—present in some vitamin and mineral supplements—taken during the second or third trimester may adversely affect the thyroid of the fetus.

Radioactive iodine, often used in the diagnosis of thyroid disorders, is absolutely contraindicated during all stages of pregnancy because it can destroy the fetal thyroid gland. For that matter, all forms of ionizing radiation, including X rays, should be avoided during all stages of pregnancy, unless a physician determines that such use warrants the possible risk of fetal damage. Rarely is pelvimetry (assessment by means of X ray of the pregnant woman's pelvis prior to delivery) needed by the obstetrician. Pelvimetry by X ray has been virtually replaced by ultrasonography, which utilizes sound waves rather than X rays. If X rays during pregnancy are absolutely necessary, rigid precautions should be enforced to minimize risk to the fetus. CU's medical consultants suggest that women who are potentially pregnant take the additional precaution, when possible, of scheduling any X-ray procedures or radioactive isotope tests during the ten days following the start of menstruation.*

There are special risks at the end of pregnancy too—and even immediately following delivery of the infant. Several antibiotics may pose hazards, ranging from mild to serious, to the fetus as well as to the newborn baby. Sulfonamides taken by the mother shortly before delivery may increase the possibility of a certain type of jaundice in the infant. The tetracycline class of broad-spectrum antibiotics (see Chapter 26) may cause permanent staining of the unerupted tooth buds of the fetus. However, for infections that can be combated only with antibiotics, penicillin remains safe for use in pregnancy—except, of course, for those allergic to that drug.

Central nervous system depressants, such as barbiturates or narcotics, can slow the breathing of the newborn baby if taken by the mother in high doses during labor and delivery. Anticoagulants, such as warfarin (Athrombin-K, Coumadin, Panwarfin), can cause excessive bleeding in both mother and infant

*Every woman of childbearing age about to undergo X-ray procedures should be asked by the physician or X-ray technician ordering or performing the X ray whether there is any possibility of pregnancy. If so, the X ray should be postponed, if possible. At the very least, protective lead shielding should be used.

at time of birth and, in some instances, facial deformities in the fetus. Use of indomethacin (Indocin) and aspirin by near-term women has been implicated as contributing to pulmonary hypertension of the newborn.

To call the roll of all the drugs now known to damage, or now suspected of damaging, the fetus and newborn baby would serve no useful purpose—and might lead to a false sense of security with respect to other drugs not yet adequately studied. Before any inclusive list can be compiled, intensive surveillance of birth defects, as well as studies of how pregnant women use drugs—both over-the-counter (OTC) and prescription—are required. Indeed, there is also a theoretical possibility that some medications taken by males may affect genetic material in sperm and thus influence fetal development. Researchers have found that a diverse group of known teratogens, when given to male animals only, cause birth defects. These teratogens include alcohol, caffeine, lead, and some narcotics. So far no one is certain how substances administered to (or taken by) males can cause birth defects. A study made at the University of Vermont discussed several possibilities. Among these were first, that drugs could directly damage sperm. And second, drugs could be carried in the semen and absorbed through the vaginal walls, thus entering the bloodstream of the female and of the developing fetus.

A special warning is warranted about the drugs commonly found in the home medicine cabinet. So generally used a drug as plain aspirin can interfere with the coagulation mechanism of both mother and baby at delivery. Aspirin in high dosage also has been associated in at least one study with an increase in the average length of pregnancy as well as the duration of normal labor. Some learning disabilities have been observed in offspring of laboratory mice given aspirin, although there is no evidence of this phenomenon in human beings. No common home remedy, even antacid preparations, should be assumed to be completely safe in terms of its possible effect on the fetus or newborn.

Vitamins have been known to cause harm to the fetus when taken in excessive doses by a pregnant woman. Vitamin C, widely publicized both as a cold treatment and as a cold preventive may possibly cause scurvy in a newborn infant if taken in high doses by the mother during pregnancy. This is due to the fact that at labor the large supply of ascorbic acid to which the infant has become accustomed—because of maternal ingestion—is suddenly stopped. High doses of pyridoxine (vitamin B_6), taken by the mother, may be associated with withdrawal seizures in the infant. Large doses of vitamin K, if administered near the delivery date, may increase the severity of jaundice in certain infants.

The hazards of excessive amounts of vitamins A and D—which exist for everyone, not just pregnant women—led the FDA in 1973 to set limits on the amounts permitted in OTC vitamin pills: 10,000 international units for vitamin A and 400 for vitamin D. Higher amounts could be obtained by prescription. The FDA statement announcing the limitation included the comment that among the disorders in which excessive amounts of these vitamins have been implicated were mental and physical retardation. CU and its medical consultants believe it to be unfortunate that this restriction was revoked by Congress in 1978.

There is some evidence that dietary deficiencies of certain nutrients such as vitamin C and folic acid may produce defects in the fetus. Many obstetricians therefore prescribe vitamins in conventional therapeutic dosages for their pregnant patients. It is important that such dosages not be exceeded, however.

A word of caution is also in order concerning medicated salves, ointments, nose drops, suppositories, vaginal creams and jellies, and similar products applied to the skin. Such topical medications may contain substances that can be absorbed through the skin into the bloodstream and thus affect fetal development. To indicate the nature of such hazards, the FDA issues guidelines for the labeling of medications. For example, the labeling suggested by the FDA for ointments containing cortisone and related steroids is: "Although topical steroids have not been reported to have an adverse effect on pregnancy, the safety of their use in pregnancy has not been established. Therefore, they should not be used extensively on pregnant patients, in large amounts or for prolonged periods of time."

Possible hazards to the fetus from the illicit use of narcotics, hallucinogens, and other mood-altering drugs are discussed in detail in another CU book, *Licit and Illicit Drugs*, by Edward M. Brecher and the Editors of Consumer Reports. The socially acceptable licit drugs, caffeine, alcohol, and nicotine, have been shown to pass the placental barrier. Studies based on animal data have implicated caffeine as a possible cause of birth defects. A study conducted by the University of Washington School of Medicine and published in 1973 established a link between maternal alcoholism and birth defects. The researchers concluded that the data point to serious fetal malformations as a possible consequence of alcoholism in the mother.

In 1977 the National Institute on Alcohol Abuse and Alcoholism warned pregnant women that more than two drinks a day (about three ounces of whiskey) may harm their unborn children. The Institute has stated that there are more than 100 studies that show a link between a pregnant woman's alcohol intake and malformed or retarded infants. Joseph Cruse, M.D., of the University of Southern California has put the risk of fetal alcohol syndrome defects at 10 percent if a woman drinks between two and four ounces of liquor daily. He recommends that pregnant women completely abstain from alcohol. The requirement for warning labels on alcoholic beverages is under consideration by the government and the Distilled Spirits Council. The warning, as recommended by the Bureau of Alcohol, Tobacco, and Firearms, would read: "Caution—Consumption of alcoholic beverages may be hazardous to your health, may be habit-forming, and may cause birth defects when consumed during pregnancy."

Pregnant cigarette smokers have had ample notice that nicotine is associated with an increased risk of fetal and infant mortality. A U.S. Public Health Service report to Congress in 1973 on health implications of smoking reviewed the available research and concluded that about 4,600 stillbirths a year in the United States could probably be attributed to smoking. The report made reference to a 1972 British study on women who smoked during pregnancy, which showed a 30 percent increased risk of stillborn children and a 26 percent higher risk of infant death within the first few days after birth. However, there is some evidence that women who are able to stop smoking by the fourth month of pregnancy decrease the risk. Smokers, authorities agree, tend to produce babies with a lower average birth weight than do nonsmokers.

An article published in 1973 in the *British Medical Journal* reported the results of a study of children born to mothers who smoked more than half a pack of cigarettes a day during the second half of their pregnancy. These children, at ages seven and eleven, were found to demonstrate a mild degree of mental and physical retardation. Richard L. Naeye, M.D., of Pennsylvania State University, head pathologist for the Collaborative Perinatal Project of the National Institute of Neurological and Communicative Disorders and Stroke, has stated that no one knows how long the effects of smoking continue after a woman quits. But he has advised women contemplating pregnancy to give up smoking.

Adequate maternal nutrition has been shown by many researchers to be of immense importance in pregnancy. It has been accepted for many years that poor nutrition results in lowered birth weights and decreased growth rates for the newborn. And larger weight gains are now recommended for pregnant women than were once thought acceptable. These findings are especially important in light of some current diet fads. CU's medical consultants strongly discourage strenuous dieting, especially low-carbohydrate regimens, during pregnancy. These may result in ketosis (the presence of ketone bodies in the blood due to incomplete burning of body fat), which has been linked with subsequent mental retardation in children born to mothers on such diets.

It is extremely difficult to detect such abnormalities as mental retardation—or behavioral defects, especially when they are minimal—and to correlate them with ingestion of substances during pregnancy. Some substances may indeed be toxic to the fetus, and these include food additives as well as drugs. Red 2, which was a widely used coloring for foods and beverages (as well as drugs and cosmetics), was judged a possible risk to the fetus, particularly in the period immediately following conception. The possibility that Red 2 might be a cancer-causing agent led the FDA in 1976 to issue a ban on its use. Saccharin is another additive that may be hazardous to pregnant women. In 1975 *The Medical Letter* warned that saccharin may accumulate in fetal tissue.

Hazards to pregnancy other than those induced by drugs or chemicals are not within the scope of this chapter. CU's medical consultants suggest one exception: A warning about toxoplasmosis. This infection, when contracted in pregnancy, may damage the brain and other organs of the fetus. There is evidence that the organism may be transmitted to the fetus when a pregnant woman eats undercooked meat, handles a cat, or tends to a cat's litter pan. Some authorities estimate that about one-third of all adults are immune to toxoplasmosis because of previous undetected infection.

Dietary practices, environmental pollutants, emotional stress—all of these may interact in such a way as to produce subtle abnormalities, some of which may not even be recognized until many years after birth. There is evidence that some serious abnormalities do indeed take years to develop. One example is the discovery of a hitherto rare type of vaginal cancer in the teenage daughters of women who took diethylstilbestrol (DES) during their pregnancies in an attempt to avert miscarriage. Special techniques are required to diagnose this uncommon form of vaginal cancer. It is undetectable by the customary Pap smear test used to diagnose cervical cancer. Any DES daughter should consult a gynecologist knowledgeable in this area. Studies of DES sons have shown nonmalignant genital abnormalities in some and evidence of impaired fertility in others.

Correlation between drug use, in its broadest sense, and possible damage to the fetus or the child requires a high degree of suspicion and vigilance on the part of practicing physicians. It also requires that they follow up on any suspected side effect or risk and report to the FDA what they believe to be an adverse drug reaction.

Many suggestions have been made by competent authorities for further reducing the risks of drugs in pregnancy. Here are five proposals CU supports.

1. *Increased understanding about drugs in pregnancy on the part of physicians and their patients.* Shortly before the thalidomide disaster, a study made in California showed an incredible number of drugs—nearly 11,000 in all—actually prescribed by physicians to 3,072 women whose pregnancies began during the year ending March 31, 1961. Only 244 of the patients (7.9

percent) went through pregnancy without a prescription; and only 563 (18.3 percent) had only one drug prescribed; 617 women received more than five drugs each, and 121 received ten or more. A few received twenty or more different drugs. These totals did not include self-prescribed drugs, OTC drugs, and drugs prescribed before pregnancy that patients continued to take during pregnancy. And keep in mind that some prescriptions can contain more than one drug ingredient. The actual number of risks was considerably higher, because one drug alone may be effective and safe but may be rendered ineffective or harmful when taken at the same time as one or more other drugs.

Some of the drugs prescribed were no doubt essential for the health or well-being of the patient or her unborn baby; but many others were probably superfluous. For example, 426 of the 3,072 women received prescriptions for medicated lotions or creams (usually for skin conditions), 716 received analgesics, 443 were prescribed antiobesity drugs or appetite suppressants, 533 received antihistamines (mostly because they had colds), 605 received barbiturates or other sedatives and hypnotics, and so on down the long list.

How much more cautious have physicians become when they write prescriptions for their pregnant patients? No one really knows. But the evidence is not encouraging. In 1971 the *British Medical Journal* published a report that more than 97 percent of the 1,369 pregnant women included in a study took drugs prescribed by their doctors, and 65 percent of them practiced self-medication. A later survey in Scotland seemed to confirm these findings. Of the 911 women included in the Scottish study, 82 percent were prescribed drugs (exclusive of iron) during pregnancy—with an average of four drugs prescribed for each woman—and 65 percent of the pregnant women dosed themselves with OTC preparations. In the

United States, a study centered in Houston (and reported to a 1973 symposium sponsored by The National Foundation–March of Dimes) revealed that each pregnant woman participating in the survey took an average of ten different drugs. One participant in the Houston study—confined to women in middle- and upper-class socioeconomic groups—who took twenty-five aspirins daily during her pregnancy reported that she would never have done so had she known aspirin was a drug.

In view of these findings, CU recommends that educational programs about drugs in pregnancy—for doctors and the general public alike—be given priority. Doctors should be strongly encouraged to consider the risks when prescribing or advising medication for a pregnant patient—or for a potentially pregnant patient. And if medication is warranted, a patient should be warned to take drugs only in prescribed amounts and for specified durations. There is urgent need for clearly worded warnings and guidelines to be prepared for distribution to pregnant women by doctors, pharmacists, clinics, and other health agencies.

2. *International cooperation in testing.* Following the thalidomide disaster, the United States, Canada, Britain, France, Germany, and other countries tightened up animal test procedures. In most respects, foreign test requirements are less strict than the FDA guidelines. In some testing programs, however, there is too much costly duplication. Substantially the same test, with only minor variations, must be run over and over again to satisfy the requirements of all the countries in which a new drug is to be marketed. If the FDA and comparable agencies in other countries could agree upon a series of test protocols, money now wasted in duplicate tests could be devoted to a far broader battery of additional tests.

The FDA has formulated guidelines under which certain

clinical drug studies performed abroad would be acceptable in this country as part of the review process preliminary to approval of any new drug application. In this way research data accumulated outside the United States would not need to be duplicated as long as the studies conform to generally recognized international standards. In a proposal filed in 1973, the FDA announced that its standards for acceptability would be based on the recommendations of the Eighteenth World Medical Assembly, which had met in Helsinki, Finland, in 1964. Fully operative, the FDA program could lead the way to increased international cooperation in testing procedures.

3. *Primate tests.* Most new-drug tests are now performed on pregnant rats, mice, and rabbits. The FDA "encourages" tests on pregnant monkeys but does not require them; they are rarely run because they are so expensive. Would tests on monkeys or other primates more closely related to humans than rats, mice, and rabbits secure results more valid for pregnant women? No one really knows; there have been too few primate tests. A large-scale research program designed to determine whether primate tests are worth the extra cost is thus CU's third recommendation.

4. *Reporting of adverse effects.* The thalidomide hazard was unmasked when physicians in West Germany and Australia noted a sudden, startling increase in infant malformations of a type encountered only rarely before. Improved procedures for reporting events of this kind have been instituted. It is unlikely that if another drug like thalidomide comes along its teratogenic effects would be overlooked until 10,000 babies had been afflicted.

But the problem has not been solved. We can hardly expect that the next teratogen to be discovered will produce such a dramatic and readily recognizable pattern of otherwise rare defects. The next new drug may produce mental retardation, for example, or premature birth or some other already common misfortune. If so, it may affect thousands of babies without revealing itself; such afflictions could easily go unnoticed among the countless similar cases already occurring. What is needed as an alerting mechanism is continuous registry of the occurrence of all malformations and other perinatal conditions in an entire population. Then, if some common condition is seen to be increasing in frequency, a search for causes can be promptly undertaken.

In 1951 the Canadian province of British Columbia developed a registry for the reporting of major birth defects; minor birth defects were also recorded beginning in 1963. Since 1977 five other provinces have joined with British Columbia in a nationally coordinated surveillance program for reporting defects detected during the first year after birth. In the United States, the first comparable program was begun in 1967 and covers metropolitan Atlanta. Six Florida counties have monitored birth defects since 1971; a program for the state of Nebraska was initiated in May 1973. However, it was not until November 1974 that the large-scale registry of birth defects began in the United States. As of 1979 about 1,200 hospitals nationwide participate in the Birth Defects Monitoring Program, which is being coordinated by the Center for Disease Control in Atlanta.

Surveillance of approximately 1 million births yearly are being based on computer data compiled from records of the participating hospitals. Limitations are built into the monitoring system, however, since hospital records of newborns may not include such information about the child's mother as age, number of previous pregnancies, and medications taken during pregnancy. Although the Canadian and United States programs would undoubtedly discover any disaster on the scale of the thalidomide tragedy, these systems probably cannot detect the causes of small clusters of birth defects. Even the more sophisticated Canadian system does not provide for the kinds of information necessary to establish a clear connection between birth defects and maternal drug use.

Authorities on surveillance of birth defects believe some relatively simple changes would improve the effectiveness of monitoring programs. Procedures for linking birth defects with maternal factors could probably be strengthened if terminology were standardized, hospital records were kept in a uniform fashion, and hospital admission records for infants required information about the mother (such as her age).

The joint effort of pediatrician Sydney S. Gellis, M.D., of Tufts University, computer expert John J. Donovan of Massachusetts Institute of Technology, and Daniel Bergsma, M.D., of The National Foundation–March of Dimes has produced a computer system that will offer physicians an extensive diagnostic and consultative service covering more than 1,400 birth defects. Physicians who have access to a computer terminal, as in many hospitals, will be able to ask the central computer at MIT about a patient's symptoms. The computer will return an answer, suggest tests, and request results. If the symptoms suggest a new syndrome, the computer will store these data.

5. *Patient package inserts.* Before any drug can be marketed, the pharmaceutical firm responsible must secure FDA approval of a "package insert" or "product information circular," which lists precautions and contraindications as well as indications, dosages, and other important data. One difficulty with package inserts as a means of alerting busy physicians to a drug's possible hazards for pregnant women has been the question of format and type size. The information about pregnancy could once have been a few words buried in a thousand words or more of small type on other subjects—an unlabeled item under "Warnings" or "Contraindications," say.

As of December 26, 1979, however, new FDA regulations for prescription drug labeling require specific information about a drug's potential for possible harm to the fetus. Listed under "Precautions," a special subsection on pregnancy is now mandated for all drugs absorbed systemically and likely to affect the fetus. Such drugs are labeled according to one of five pregnancy categories: A, B, C, D, or X.

A. The possibility of fetal harm is remote. Adequate and well-controlled studies in pregnant women have shown no increase in risk of fetal abnormalities.

B. The possibility of fetal harm appears remote. Either animal tests have failed to demonstrate a risk to the fetus and there have been no human studies, or animal studies have shown some evidence of risk, but well-controlled tests with pregnant women have provided contrary evidence.

C. Benefits outweigh potential risks. Either there have been no animal or human studies demonstrating adverse effects, or animal studies have shown teratogenic effects but there have been no adequate and well-controlled studies in humans.

D. There is potential hazard to the fetus. Positive evidence of risks based on adverse reactions in humans must be weighed against potential benefit from the drug.

X. Fetal abnormalities have been demonstrated.

Labeling must also include information on the drug's non-teratogenic effects, labor and delivery, and nursing mothers.

All the above regulations about improving package inserts deal with material addressed to physicians. CU believes that patients have a right to direct access to information about the implications of drug usage. Among the prescription drugs for which manufacturers include FDA-approved package inserts prepared especially for patients are isoproterenol (a spray used for asthma); insulin (for use in diabetes); and oral and inject-able contraceptives. In general, CU endorses this practice and would like to see it extended to cover other medications, starting with those likely to be hazardous during pregnancy. Motivated by patient injuries from drugs and pressure from consumer groups, Congress is considering two bills to provide the patient with drug information. Bills introduced by Congressman Paul D. Rogers of Florida and Senator Edward M. Kennedy of Massachusetts would require that patients be provided drug information with all prescriptions filled for them by a pharmacist.

We have stressed the drug factor in malformations and other problems of fetuses and newborn babies because something can be done about it right now, both by patients and by the medical profession. But it is also important to keep the drug factor in proper perspective.

The great majority of malformations and other unfortunate outcomes of pregnancy are caused by factors other than drugs. Even those California women who received as many as twenty drugs each during pregnancy for the most part delivered healthy babies. However, 175 of the 1,369 mothers in the British study gave birth to infants with major congenital abnormalities during the study period. But the number involved is not the only crucial factor. Drug hazards should not be stressed because the ill effects are so numerous or so likely to occur, but because when they do occur they can in some cases be so devastating. And in most instances, the hazards of drug taking can be easily avoided. Pregnant women who follow CU's precautions, listed below, and whose physicians use ordinary prudence in prescribing for their patients, can be assured that the risks and side effects of drugs in pregnancy can be minimized.

CU's medical consultants recommend that the following cautions be observed by pregnant women, as well as by fertile women who engage in sexual intercourse without contraception and who wish to become pregnant.

- No chemical has been proved to be entirely harmless for all pregnant women and their unborn babies during all stages of pregnancy. Therefore, do not take any drug unless there is a specific medical need for it. Be especially careful in the first trimester of pregnancy and just before delivery.

- If there *is* a medical need, and if your physician prescribes a drug to meet that need, take it only in the amounts and at the times specified. Do not increase or reduce the dose; do not discontinue usage sooner or continue it longer than directed. Remember that your unborn baby's health can be adversely affected by your failure to take a needed drug, as well as by your indulgence in unprescribed medication.

- A number of drugs exert their adverse effects during the first weeks following a missed menstrual period—the weeks when you are likely to be wondering whether you are pregnant. Therefore, if pregnancy is a possibility, discontinue all self-prescribed remedies within a few days after an expected menstrual period fails to occur, and recheck with your doctor concerning drugs previously prescribed for you. If you are trying to become pregnant, be sure to tell your doctor this if a drug is prescribed for you.

- During pregnancy and also during the time you may wish to become pregnant, curtail the use of OTC "home remedies," as well as drugs available only on a doctor's prescription.* Even common self-prescribed medicines, such as aspirin, should be taken sparingly—except on your doctor's advice.

---

*Mothers who breast-feed their babies should continue to avoid the use of medications as much as possible. Numerous drugs taken by the mother are excreted in her milk and reach the nursing baby. If a nursing mother is prescribed a medication by her personal physician, she should tell the doctor that she is breast-feeding her baby.

▪ Interpret the term "drugs" broadly to include many things besides oral preparations and injections—for example, lotions and ointments containing hormones or other drugs that may be absorbed through the skin, and vaginal douches, suppositories, and jellies.

23

Estrogen replacement therapy

Promotional campaigns for estrogen replacement therapy started in the 1960s and, fed by the preachings of a few physicians, flourished for more than a decade. Many menopausal and postmenopausal women were tantalized by the promise that they could remain healthy, youthful, and attractive for the rest of their lives. The promise was summed up in the slogan "Feminine Forever," which was also the title of the book that helped spark the estrogen boom.

Menopause, which typically begins in the mid-to-late forties, is commonly defined as the cessation of regular menstrual periods. It is caused by the gradual decline of estrogen production by the ovaries. Menopause is not a hormone-deficiency disease; it is a normal stage of life. (Some premenopausal women, for medical reasons, undergo removal of both ovaries; they experience "surgical menopause," the result of the abrupt elimination of the body's major source of estrogen.)

Estrogen replacement has been prescribed by physicians for more than thirty-five years to afford women relief from the sometimes distressing symptoms of menopause. But the use of estrogens—particularly in their most frequently prescribed form, called conjugated estrogens—nearly tripled between

1965 and 1975. Millions of menopausal women without severe symptoms were encouraged to take the drug routinely as a cure-all for aging, for the degenerative diseases associated with aging, and for the emotional difficulties purportedly linked with middle age. Estrogen replacement therapy grew into an $80 million-a-year bonanza for the drug industry.

But then reports of another side to estrogen therapy began to circulate: Instead of maintaining health and prolonging life, long-term use of estrogen replacement reportedly caused cancer of the endometrium (the lining of the uterus), and there was also some evidence that the therapy might increase the risk of cancer of the breast as well as cardiovascular diseases—heart attack, stroke, hypertension, and thromboembolism—and gallbladder disease. For many women the dream of agelessness through drug therapy turned into a nightmare of fear and dread. Some simply stopped taking estrogens on their own. Others, on the advice of their physicians, reduced dosages or tried another dosage form of the drug (for example, in a vaginal cream rather than in pill form) or, most commonly, abandoned estrogens altogether. Some women remained on estrogen therapy, and some who had quit returned to it, because for them the benefits were worth the reported risks.

For some women estrogen therapy can be of substantial benefit in relieving certain menopausal symptoms. However, there has been almost as much medical controversy about the advantages of treatment as about the hazards. Much of the controversy centers on the nature of menopause itself.

Women usually begin menstruating at about age thirteen (some start as early as ten, others by sixteen). Menstruation continues at fairly regular intervals, normally as long as the ovaries provide adequate levels of estrogen. Estrogen levels exert a variety of other effects on the body, including maintenance of secondary sex characteristics and normal vaginal lubrication. It is rare for a women to be younger than forty or older than fifty-five when menopause begins.

If the cessation of menstruation were the only consequence of a decline in the body's estrogen levels, few women would feel the need to seek medical assistance and take costly medication. In fact, some women experience little or no distress during and after menopause, while others experience acute distress.

Although recent evidence has shown that progressive bone loss occurs with menopause, hot flashes and vaginal atrophy are the primary physical manifestations distinctly characteristic of menopause—other than cessation of menstrual periods. About 50 percent of menopausal women experience hot flashes; virtually every woman will eventually develop vaginal atrophy to some degree.

What makes some women more vulnerable to menopausal symptoms than others? The extent and the rate of decline of estrogen production by the ovaries vary from woman to woman and may affect the severity of symptoms. Contrary to the reasoning of "Feminine Forever" enthusiasts, however, "estrogen starvation" does not usually follow on the heels of menopause. The adrenal glands continue to supply the body with small amounts of estrogen that may help to cushion the fall in the ovaries' production of estrogen. Estrogen can also continue to be made after menopause from an adrenal hormone by enzymes in the body's fat cells. With some women, the ovaries themselves continue low-level estrogen production for many years beyond menopause.

There is no question that menopause is dramatic and undeniable evidence of aging and of the loss of reproductive capability—a double blow for some in a society that has traditionally emphasized the desirability of youth, good looks, and sexuality for everyone—and reproduction and child care for women. Yet, despite physical manifestations of the aging process, femininity need not decline as hormones decline and sexuality need not diminish. Whether in response to their perceived change in status or to hormonal changes, some menopausal women experience a cluster of psychological symptoms. They may feel nervous, tired, or dejected. They may be plagued by quick mood changes, laughing one minute and crying the next. They may suffer from insomnia. How much these emotional manifestations are associated with hormonal changes generally or with the specific distress of hot flashes or vaginal atrophy is not known.

Some menopausal women have hot flashes to a disabling degree. With a hot flash, a wave of heat, lasting from a few seconds to a few minutes, spreads over the chest, neck, and/or head. It is usually accompanied by a "flush," or increased reddening, and sometimes by drenching sweats. Flashes can occur as often as ten to twenty times a day. They may be responsible for sleeplessness, fatigue, and irritability. A woman may experience such flashes for only a few months, or they may continue for years. In most cases, they cease within a year or two. With some women, hot flashes may recur years later, usually at times of particular stress.

So far, the precise cause of hot flashes has eluded investigators, but research into changes in skin temperature and blood chemistry during episodes of hot flashes has provided evidence that this symptom is a biologically measurable event and not "just in your head."

Atrophy of the vaginal lining of postmenopausal women is a direct consequence of lowered levels of naturally produced estrogens. Usually this condition does not fully develop until a decade or two after menstruation ceases, but it can begin sooner. With menopause, vaginal secretions and lubrication may decrease, the vaginal lining begins to thin, and the vagina may become less elastic. Symptoms such as itching, burning, and pain during intercourse may accompany these changes. Urinary discomfort may also occur.

While dosage may vary from woman to woman, it is clear that estrogen therapy can alleviate hot flashes and vaginal atrophy.

The benefits and risks for menopausal and postmenopausal women of treating these symptoms with estrogen therapy was the subject considered in September 1979 at a two-day Consensus Development Conference sponsored by the National Institute on Aging of the National Institutes of Health (NIH). Its purpose: To assemble what was known and not known about estrogen therapy. Participants included biomedical research scientists, practicing physicians, representatives of women's interest groups and consumer organizations, and others concerned with efficacy and safety of estrogen therapy.

In a comprehensive review of the benefits of estrogen replacement prepared for the NIH Consensus Development Conference, Isaac Schiff, M.D., and Kenneth J. Ryan, M.D. (of Boston Hospital for Women, Harvard Medical School), pointed out that hot flashes, even without therapy, lessen with time. "In contrast," they stated, "vaginal atrophy progressively worsens. If the patient is sexually active she may complain of both vaginal dryness and pain with intercourse. Unfortunately, some women are reluctant to discuss this with their physicians; and at the same time some physicians feel ill at ease in bringing up sexual matters with older patients. The silence that may enshroud this problem is all the sadder in that sexual intercourse may remain an important part of the life of the aging woman. The symptoms of [painful intercourse] may respond very dramatically to estrogen therapy."

As for the psychological symptoms experienced by some menopausal women, "There is no evidence at present to justify the use of estrogens in treatment of primary psychological problems," the NIH Consensus Development Conference report stated. The report added that studies have shown some improvement in sleep or in emotional well-being among women taking estrogens but suggested that such improvement may have been a secondary result of the alleviation of hot flashes and/or vaginal atrophy.

Women who experience *severe* psychological difficulty at menopause have probably experienced emotional problems prior to menopause. "Menopause by itself does not induce depression, but in a depressive person, menopause will bring out a depression," according to Marvin Fogel, M.D., of the Mount Sinai Medical Center in New York. "Emotionally, it acts as a trigger for what is there already."

"Feminine Forever" advocates have prescribed long-term estrogen replacement to promote a youthful appearance and to stave off the degenerative diseases of aging. But aging is governed by such factors as heredity and health. According to medical authorities, estrogen replacement cannot prevent or reverse the aging process. For example, estrogen treatment cannot retard the wrinkling of skin, nor is there proof that it can lengthen life.

Still another claim for estrogen replacement is that it can prevent or delay coronary artery disease. Several surveys have shown that men in their thirties and forties develop coronary artery disease much more frequently than women. The gap narrows in the fifties, and, after sixty, women catch up with men. Could it be that high levels of naturally produced estrogens provide some protection to premenopausal women, protection that declines with the fall in estrogen production?

That suggestion has been put aside. The current medical belief is that there is no sudden increase in heart disease in women after menopause, but rather a steady increase with advancing age. According to current thinking, there is a particular, but still undefined, group of *men* who are vulnerable to premature coronary disease. It is that group that accounts for the statistical difference in heart attacks between younger men and premenopausal women.

Still unresolved is the advisability of using estrogen replacement to treat and prevent osteoporosis—the thinning and increased porosity of bone—and to prevent bone fractures. About one out of four postmenopausal women eventually suffers from a serious form of osteoporosis. It commonly produces backache and may involve a decrease in size of one or more of the back bones leading to a shortening or bending of the spine (the so-called dowager's hump). Osteoporosis may also result in hip and wrist fractures. Usually diagnosed by X ray as a generalized decrease in density of the skeleton, osteoporosis is but one of several diseases that can produce a similar radiological appearance. These diseases include calcium and vitamin D deficiencies, parathyroid gland overactivity, and certain cancers. At times, diagnosis may be difficult; occasionally bone biopsy may be necessary.

Osteoporosis has been linked to lowered estrogen levels because its incidence increases after menopause. The disease develops sooner and more severely in young women who experience early surgical menopause and who do not take estrogens. Occasionally osteoporosis can occur in young women with normal estrogen levels. And three out of four postmenopausal women remain free of the severe variety of the disease. Why some postmenopausal women become more osteoporotic than others is not known. Both groups may be equally estrogen-deficient. Estrogen deficiency is only one factor associated with osteoporosis. Other possible factors are physical inactivity, calcium and protein deficiency, and general malnutrition.

In addition to estrogen replacement, the treatment of the pain of osteoporosis may involve other therapeutic approaches, some of them still experimental, including calcium, fluoride, vitamin D, calcitonin (a hormone causing calcium to be deposited in bone), a high-protein diet, and exercise.

What about estrogen use for *preventing* osteoporosis—probably the most commonly given medical rationale for long-term estrogen therapy in postmenopausal women. One of the main reasons for prescribing estrogen replacement therapy for women who experience early surgical menopause is the prevention of osteoporosis. Clinical studies have shown that estrogen therapy prevents bone loss (measured by accurate analyses of bone density); these studies appear to be well documented. The evidence that such therapy actually prevents fractures is only suggestive. In addition, the use of estrogen, once the bone loss process has begun, may halt the loss, but affected bone will not be restored to normal. When estrogen replacement therapy is stopped, bone loss resumes at its former rate. However, even with interrupted estrogen use some degree of protection against future fractures may take place. The NIH Concensus Development Conference called for more research in the area. Apparently what is needed is some method of identifying which women are at high risk of developing severe postmenopausal osteoporosis and resultant fractures. Treatment of such a target population might improve the benefit-to-risk ratio of postmenopausal estrogen use.

In late 1978 the Food and Drug Administration (FDA) officially recognized that estrogens are effective in preventing bone loss in postmenopausal women. Adolphe T. Gregoire, Ph.D., executive secretary of the FDA's endocrine and metabolism advisory committee, stated that although the committee accepted the evidence that estrogens retard bone loss, the decision to prescribe the drug will be up to individual physicians, who must weigh the presumed benefits against the current warnings about the association of the hormone with cancer.

The foregoing sums up the "state of the art" insofar as the

purported benefits of estrogen replacement therapy are concerned. Now what of the risks—in particular the risk of cancer?

In a review prepared for the NIH Consensus Development Conference, Barbara S. Hulka, M.D., professor of epidemiology at the University of North Carolina, reported on eight case-control studies of the association of endometrial cancer with postmenopausal estrogen use. The studies, dating from 1975, indicated that menopausal women who use estrogen replacement therapy are more likely to develop cancer of the endometrium than are menopausal women who do not use such therapy. (Of course, women who undergo hysterectomy —removal of the uterus—are not at risk.)

In Seattle, the histories of 317 patients with endometrial cancer—some estrogen users, some nonusers—were compared with the estrogen replacement histories of 317 women with other forms of cancer. From the results, the investigators calculated that users of estrogen replacement were 4.5 times more likely to develop endometrial cancer than nonusers.

A study of women enrolled in a Los Angeles prepaid medical-care plan uncovered the same trend. After reviewing the histories of 94 women with endometrial cancer and 188 without, the researchers calculated that the risk of endometrial cancer was 7.6 times greater for those who used conjugated estrogens than for the nonusers. The risk grew with duration of use. For women who took estrogen replacement for seven or more years, it was 13.9 times greater than for nonusers.

In a third independent study, conducted at a California retirement community, women who had used estrogen replacement were found to be eight times more likely to develop endometrial cancer than nonusers. The degree of risk appeared to increase with the dose.

The scientific validity of these retrospective studies was questioned by Ralph I. Horwitz, M.D., and Alvan R. Feinstein, M.D., of the Yale University School of Medicine. In late 1978 they called attention to the possibility of a built-in bias which, if true, might overestimate the incidence of endometrial carcinoma in estrogen users. They pointed out that postmenopausal women who experience vaginal bleeding while taking estrogen replacement therapy receive increased diagnostic attention; therefore their cancer is detected earlier than in women not using the medication. The women who were not on hormone treatment might not have the bleeding that would alert their physicians to perform the necessary investigation.

The Horwitz-Feinstein study has been challenged by other researchers who maintain that, although estrogen users may have their cancer diagnosed somewhat earlier, virtually all women with endometrial cancer ultimately will have the disease diagnosed, and thus even if screening advances the date of diagnosis, it should have little effect on the total number of cases ultimately discovered.

In January 1979, Paul D. Stolley, M.D., and Carlos M. F. Antunes, Sc.D., and their co-investigators reported in *The New England Journal of Medicine* on a study of 1,339 menopausal women. They concluded that those who were given estrogen replacement therapy were six times more likely than nonusers to have cancer of the uterus. For those who used the medication for more than five years the risk was found to be fifteen times greater. The researchers used methodology that compensated for the possible bias brought forth by the Horwitz-Feinstein study and concluded that the use of estrogen replacement therapy still appeared to have a statistically significant risk of uterine cancer attached to it. They cautioned that patients who receive replacement therapy be monitored regularly, by procedures that sample the uterine lining, to detect early asymptomatic cancer.

In February 1979, *The New England Journal of Medicine*

reported on a study by the Boston Collaborative Drug Surveillance Program, which bolstered the conclusion that long-term users of estrogens are at considerably higher risk for endometrial cancer than those not using estrogens. The report also stated that discontinuation of hormone therapy is followed by a rapid decline in that risk.

Although the recent retrospective studies do not prove that estrogen replacement therapy *causes* endometrial cancer, they do indicate a strong association between the two—an association consistent with animal studies and human biology. The association is also consistent with a reported rise in endometrial cancer rates in eight areas of the United States. For a time, the incidence of endometrial cancer was reportedly increasing in some areas at a rate of 10 percent a year—an "increase in incidence of a magnitude that has rarely been paralleled in the history of cancer reporting in this country," said the research team headed by Noel Weiss, M.D., of the University of Washington, Seattle. In general, the increase was greatest in women fifty years old or older who were in high socioeconomic groups —the women most likely to be using estrogen replacement therapy. Further confirmation of the association has come from epidemiologists who found that the number of prescriptions written for estrogens paralleled the rise in incidence of endometrial cancer—until 1976, when adverse publicity about the safety of estrogen replacement became widespread. Since then the incidence of endometrial cancer and the number of estrogen prescriptions have declined in parallel.

According to Weiss, the normal risk of endometrial cancer in postmenopausal women with an intact uterus is one case per thousand women per year. But with regular use of estrogen replacement therapy, the risk grows to four to eight cases per thousand per year.

Hulka commented on two aspects of the data involving

estrogen replacement therapy and endometrial cancer—the so-called latency period and recency period. Latency period refers to the time interval from the *start* of drug use until the date of cancer diagnosis. Recency period refers to the interval between *last* use of the drug and the date of cancer diagnosis. In the case of estrogen replacement and endometrial cancer, both latency and recency were relatively brief. Latency was about two to four years. As for recency, "On average, a two-year estrogen-free interval is sufficient to eliminate any excess risk of endometrial cancer," Hulka said. "For the withdrawal of a presumed carcinogen, this represents a very short time interval for risks to drop to non-user levels. After five years of abstinence, ex-smokers only reduce their risk of lung cancer by one-half, which is still far greater than the risk for non-smokers." Hulka noted that the short latency and recency intervals suggest that estrogen acts as a promotional agent for cancer rather than as a direct cause of cancer.

The NIH conference report confirmed that the risk of endometrial cancer is four to eight times greater after two to four years of estrogen use. According to Hulka, "The finding of increasing endometrial cancer risk with increasing duration of estrogen use is the most consistent finding from all reported studies."

The conference report also pointed out that estrogen use was most commonly associated with the lowest grade and earliest stage of endometrial cancer, and that while the incidence of the disease rose, mortality from the disease did not increase. "A considerable part of this discrepancy may be attributable to early detection and the high cure rate," the report stated.

Endometrial cancer may not be the only malignancy associated with the use of estrogen replacement by postmenopausal women. A possible link with breast cancer—the leading cause of cancer death in women in the United States

—is also of concern. The evidence, however, remains inconclusive.

According to Hulka, "The preponderance of evidence from well designed case-control studies shows no increased risk of breast cancer associated with [estrogen therapy] . . . . If a decisive breast cancer risk due to estrogen existed, it should have been manifest through these multiple studies." Yet, Hulka went on, "breast tissue is hormonally dependent and it is not unreasonable to suppose that . . . estrogen would have an effect upon it. Epidemiologic studies alone have not been able to characterize this effect."

Some studies even suggest that estrogen replacement may protect against breast cancer. One such study observed that women using estrogen replacement for menopausal symptoms were at reduced risk from breast cancer during the first nine postmenopausal years, after which the protective effect was lost. Other studies, however, found the risk of breast cancer to be greater mainly during the fifth to ninth postmenopausal years of use—after which the risk dropped markedly.

The NIH conference report stated that "the association of estrogens and breast cancer in experimental animals is well known. Careful review . . . has not revealed such a relationship in humans." One study, the report said, showed an excess of breast cancer cases "only after 15 years of estrogen use." The report pointed out that "rates of breast cancer have not changed in parallel with those of estrogen use, as have those of endometrial carcinoma. Because of the high incidence and relatively poor prognosis of breast cancer, any possible association with estrogen use remains a concern."

As for the risk of cancer of the ovaries, Hulka reported that "there are no adequate epidemiologic data to support an association between estrogen use and ovarian cancer."

Among other suspected hazards of estrogen replacement

therapy have been hypertension and the increase of blood lipids and certain bloodclotting factors, which could increase the risk of potential for heart attack and stroke. "The evidence relating postmenopausal estrogen to hypertension," Hulka reported, "is, at present, mixed." The NIH conference report stated: "There is no convincing evidence that estrogens in customary doses increase the risk of thromboembolic phenomena, stroke, or heart disease in women who have undergone natural menopause." Also laid to rest was the previously held belief that estrogen replacement therapy affords postmenopausal women protection against heart attack. On the other hand, there is good evidence that postmenopausal estrogen users who smoke cigarettes will have an increased risk of heart attack. Women who may for various reasons elect to be estrogen users should be advised not to smoke.

Another association that has been noted by the Boston Collaborative group is the increased risk of developing gallbladder disease requiring surgical removal of this organ.

As with all drugs, estrogen therapy can cause other significant, if less hazardous, side effects. These include nausea, vomiting, abdominal cramps, bloating, headache, dizziness, water retention, breast engorgement and tenderness, and increase in the size of preexisting fibroids (benign tumors of the uterus).

In October 1976, the FDA proposed changes in estrogen drug labeling that would spell out for physicians the acceptable uses of estrogen replacement therapy, warn about the risk of endometrial cancer, and suggest the least hazardous treatment regimen for specific menopausal symptoms. The FDA has also prepared a package insert for patients, which manufacturers are required to provide to retailers for distribution. The American College of Obstetricians and Gynecologists (ACOG) issued a technical bulletin to physicians in October 1976, which in its summary suggested "the exercise of caution in the regular evaluation of the patient's health status and need for estrogen" but stated that no firm conclusions could be made as yet about the cancer-causing potential of estrogen replacement therapy. One physician who is a director of the ACOG advised using estrogen replacement only to treat vasomotor symptoms (like hot flashes and sweats) and vaginal atrophy. Even then, he suggested using the lowest possible dose and stopping treatment after six months to see if symptoms recur.

Ironically, the studies that elicited governmental and professional cautions were also used as a sales tool by some estrogen manufacturers. Because those studies either implicated the most widely used brand of natural conjugated estrogens—Premarin, made by Ayerst Laboratories—or did not mention specific products, some producers of other products used in estrogen replacement took heart, and advantage. Their advertisements seemed to suggest that their synthesized products, unlike natural conjugated estrogens (which are commonly derived from animal sources), were unrelated to increased cancer risk. For example, one ad for a synthetic conjugated estrogen product—Genisis, made by Organon, Inc.—heralded the "End of the age of 'natural' estrogens" and "The dawn of a new age." An ad for a synthetic single estrogen—Mead Johnson's Estrace—called the product "the major *human* estrogen . . . primary estrogen of the human ovary. . . ."

However, as Schiff and Ryan reported at the NIH conference, "There is no evidence that one form of estrogen is any more carcinogenic than another. There is no evidence that any one form of estrogen is safer than another."

In that connection, the NIH conference report referred to the common practice of using estrogen-containing cream to treat vaginal atrophy symptoms in the belief that the possible side effects of oral administration might be avoided. The report warned that "evidence now exists that the estrogens in these creams may be absorbed rapidly into the bloodstream. The biological consequences of this absorption are undetermined and require study."

Recommendations

With the evidence linking estrogen use to an increased risk of endometrial cancer as well as other potential and real hazards, caution has become the key consideration. Certain general principles are emerging, however. All women, including those who are candidates for estrogen replacement, should be aware of these principles.

Before a woman starts on estrogen replacement, for whatever reasons, her physician should take a careful history and perform a thorough physical examination. Liver disease, breast or endometrial cancer, hypertension, or heart disease would rule out estrogen replacement therapy. The physical examination should include a Pap smear for detection of cancer of the cervix. The NIH report recommended suction curettage of the uterus (to check for the presence of endometrial cancer) prior to the start of estrogen therapy. Some doctors also use a smear from the vaginal wall as an index of a woman's estrogen blood level and thereafter as a periodic check of the effectiveness of estrogen replacement therapy. A woman's symptoms may be used as well to determine the lowest effective dose, and the proper time to stop treatment.

The estrogen regimen that appears least hazardous, according to the FDA, is "cyclic administration of the lowest effective dose for the shortest possible time with appropriate monitoring for endometrial cancer." If estrogen is prescribed, it is usually given orally for twenty-one days and then withheld for seven days. That week off medication prevents continuous estrogenic stimulation of the uterus and minimizes some undesirable minor side effects, such as breast tenderness and bloating. If bleeding occurs, it generally begins toward the end of the week without treatment. Such bleeding is known as estrogen withdrawal bleeding and is similar to bleeding following the same pattern of use with some oral contraceptives. Some doctors prescribe synthetic progesterone for estrogen patients to ensure complete shedding of the endometrium. (Progesterone is a hormone produced by the ovaries in women with normal menstrual cycles. Synthetic forms of this hormone, known as progestins, are used in oral contraceptives.) But the risks and benefits of the estrogen-progesterone regimen as replacement therapy have not been adequately investigated.

Whatever the regimen, all patients on estrogen replacement should be examined by a doctor regularly, usually at six- to twelve-month intervals. Most authorities agree that an annual suction curettage of the uterus is indicated. The physician should note the effectiveness of treatment and perhaps adjust the dose. An estrogen-treated patient who experiences unscheduled vaginal bleeding should see her physician as soon as possible. Irregular menstrual bleeding during estrogen replacement therapy (or any postmenopausal bleeding) always requires evaluation because such abnormal bleeding may signal cancer. To rule out a uterine malignancy, a diagnostic curettage must be performed.

Because of the risks associated with estrogen replacement, Consumers Union's medical consultants advise that therapy be reevaluated and discontinued periodically to see if symptoms return. Vasomotor symptoms, such as hot flashes, usually need to be treated only for a period of months, according to the FDA, and rarely for longer than a year. Vaginal atrophy may require treatment for a much longer time.

The decision to use estrogen replacement therapy should not be the sole decision of the physician. If a woman is already taking estrogens, or if her doctor or an acquaintance suggests beginning estrogen replacement, she can help protect her health by being informed, being wary, and heeding the following advice.

- If a woman is now using estrogen replacement, she should ask her physician whether a trial period without the drug would be advisable for her. If the decision is to continue replacement therapy, perhaps a lower dose would still control her symptoms. Such a reevaluation would be particularly useful if she has been on estrogen replacement longer than a year; she should not think that, having been on therapy for so long, the damage is already done and there's no use going off. Endometrial cancer studies have revealed that the increased risk of cancer was lowered to normal risk levels within about two years after stopping the medication.

- A woman should not begin estrogen therapy without carefully weighing what it can do *for* her against what it can do *to* her. Because of the potential hazards, only certain symptoms warrant its use. Are her hot flashes incapacitating or diminishing quality of life? Are vaginal problems interfering with sexual activity? Is her back pain due to osteoporosis? These questions must be answered individually and the answers will depend on patient and physician attitudes.

- If it is decided that estrogen replacement is essential, request the lowest effective dose. If therapy requires regular medication, ask if a cyclic regimen—giving the body a respite from estrogen stimulation—can be prescribed.

- During estrogen therapy, periodic examinations (blood pressure, breast exam, pelvic exam, routine blood count, blood lipids, liver function tests, etc.) are essential to monitor the effects of the drug, to decide whether the dose should be changed, and to evaluate the need for continuing therapy. If a year goes by on medication and the physician has not suggested a trial period off medication—suggest it. If there is vaginal bleeding at any time other than that scheduled for withdrawal bleeding, inform the doctor at once.

- A woman should participate as a partner with her physician in considering whether estrogen replacement should be started and how it should proceed. And be sure the doctor explains the risks associated with treatment as well as the benefits that can be expected. Despite the wealth of accumulated data on the risks and benefits of estrogen replacement therapy, many questions remain unanswered.

What about the risk-to-benefit ratio of chronic estrogen use for ongoing and persistent postmenopausal changes such as osteoporosis or vaginal atrophy? How long term is long-term treatment? Does intermittent use of postmenopausal estrogen therapy prevent bone fractures without increasing the risk of endometrial cancer? Does use of a progestin in conjunction with cyclical estrogen use decrease the endometrial cancer risk? But how safe are the progestins?

In addition, a particular group deserves special attention— the premenopausal women who, for various medical indications, have had surgical removal of both ovaries at a relatively early age, ten years or more before the time of natural menopause. If these women are to lessen the risk of premature osteoporosis, vaginal atrophy, and hot flashes, they must take estrogen replacement therapy. Because of the relatively long time that such women must remain on estrogen replacement therapy, special studies of them as a group, apart from nonsurgical postmenopausal women, are clearly needed.

Just as the severity of menopausal symptoms may vary, so too does their need for treatment. CU's medical consultants believe that quality-of-life determinations should make the need for therapy a decision that should emerge from a knowledgeable and frank physician-patient interrelationship.

24
Insomnia and anxiety

At one time or another, almost everyone experiences difficulty in falling asleep or staying asleep—the two principal problems generally identified as "insomnia." Sometimes such sleep disturbances may seem transient and of no importance. But often people are moved to "take something." That something may be as innocuous as a glass of warm milk; more often, it may be a drink containing alcohol. Or a so-called hypnotic (sleep-inducing) drug obtained on prescription or an over-the-counter (OTC) product may be taken. And some people may resort to a combination of remedies to assure a good night's sleep.

What are the facts about insomnia, and just how safe and effective are the various drugs used for it?

The body's need for sleep varies widely from person to person, ranging from as little as four hours to as much as ten. From infancy, children show marked variation in sleep habits and needs. Newborns spend about eighteen hours a day asleep, on average. Investigators in Rochester, Minnesota, studied the sleep habits of a group of 783 children, aged two to three. They discovered that the total number of hours slept in a twenty-four-hour period ranged from as few as eight to as many as seventeen; the average was thirteen hours. An occasional interruption in the usual sleep pattern of a child did not result in physical or psychological harm.

Patterns of sleep begin to emerge as an individual passes through puberty into adolescence and early adulthood. School schedules, work habits, social attitudes, and even eating behavior help to create "day people," "night people," and many who go to sleep because "it's time to."

As they get older, some people find they just can't seem to sleep as well as they used to. Older people may sleep fewer hours and, just as the quantity of sleep tends to change with age, so can the quality. Older people tend to spend more of the night in light sleep with less time spent in sleeping deeply and in dreaming. Their sleep may be fitful and punctuated by frequent awakenings.

Occasional or mild difficulty in sleeping may be the result of various causes. A dripping faucet, a barking dog, or a room that's too hot or too cold may be noticed while lying awake, but rarely are they the cause of sleeplessness. Worrying over personal problems—a part of everyone's life—is often to blame. Excessive intake of caffeine, a stimulant—in beverages such as coffee, tea, cocoa, or cola drinks, or in OTC tablets such as *Excedrin, NoDoz,* and others—can contribute to sleep disturbances. Also capable of spoiling sleep are certain prescription drugs, including dextroamphetamine (Dexedrine) or methylphenidate (Ritalin), sometimes used to combat depression, and appetite-suppressant drugs sometimes used for short-term treatment of obesity, such as diethylpropion (Tenuate) and phenmetrazine (Preludin). Decongestants such as pseudoephedrine and phenylpropanolamine (the latter is also used as an OTC appetite suppressant) can interfere with sleep if taken too close to bedtime.

There is more reason for concern over severe persistent insomnia—difficulty in either falling asleep or remaining asleep almost every night. In some cases, it may be due to a physical disorder or disease. In the past few years the Stanford University Sleep Disorders Clinic has found that some insomniacs studied at the clinic were suffering from specific disturbances such as sleep apnea (temporary absence of breathing), nocturnal myoclonus (frequent muscle spasms), or from depression. In one study at the clinic, approximately half of the insomniacs under investigation were found to have various diagnosable conditions. Insomnia may be related to an underlying illness—such as heart, lung, or prostate disease—which may involve nocturnal pain, breathlessness, wheezing, coughing, or the need to awaken frequently to urinate. Successful treatment of the illness could relieve the patient of such symptoms causing insomnia.

Often chronic insomnia is a symptom of anxiety. Some people look to psychotherapy to alleviate their insomnia and the underlying anxiety. Most people, however, turn to self-treatment or are treated by their personal physician with sedatives or tranquilizers.

Among popular methods of self-treatment for persistent insomnia are a warm bath; a hot toddy; a glass of wine; various mechanical devices, such as a special mattress, a bed light, ear plugs, and eye shade; redecorating the bedroom; and listening to recordings of soothing, monotonous music, or of the hypnotic voice of a "psychologist" who, with lulling words, phrases, sounds, and rituals, attempts to help insomniacs control their anxious psyche. Unfortunately, these methods usually don't help chronic insomniacs. Some traditional remedies—such as that bedtime cup of cocoa, containing caffeine—may even inhibit sleep.

For many years insomnia was treated by physicians with alcohol (a "nightcap") or with sleeping potions containing either chloral hydrate (knockout drops when combined with alcohol) or paraldehyde, which were among the earliest drugs found to depress the central nervous system—the standard approach to sleep inducement. Alcohol does make many people relaxed and sleepy. But, because it is metabolized very quickly, alcohol often doesn't increase the total amount of sleep for the night. And as the effect of alcohol wears off, sleep often becomes disturbed, so that the drinking itself can be a cause of sleep problems. Generally, both prescription sleep medications and alcohol reduce the amount of time spent dreaming, and withdrawal from chronic use of either can lead to what is called rebound or withdrawal insomnia: Dreaming is intense, sleep is often disturbed, and nightmares may disrupt sleep further. Patients may then go back on the medication— or alcohol—and the cycle is repeated. For some people, deep sleep virtually disappears for months after they stop drinking.

Chloral hydrate, in clinical use since the nineteenth century, has relatively few side effects. But tolerance and physical dependence can occur, and gastric irritation is common if the drug is taken on an empty stomach. Thus, when barbiturates —which are also central nervous system depressants—became available early in this century, the medical profession adopted them for patient care. As hypnotics, barbiturates—especially the short-to-intermediate-acting ones such as pentobarbital (Nembutal) and secobarbital (Seconal)—are among the most effective sleep aids. As with alcohol, however, regular and prolonged use of barbiturates carries with it some risk of addiction as well as a decrease in effectiveness.

What's more, barbiturates can decrease the effectiveness of other drugs, such as anticoagulants. In addition, barbiturates can be dangerous, and even lethal in acute overdose, especially if taken together with alcohol or other drugs in the sedative or tranquilizer class. Treatment of insomnia with barbiturates or with any similar drug should be supervised by a physician, and the need for continued use reviewed periodically. Indeed, the Food and Drug Administration (FDA) has placed barbiturates —and many other central nervous system depressants and stimulants—on the list of controlled substances in an attempt to restrict nonmedical use.* Being listed limits the duration of the prescription and the number of refills, and requires that records be kept on production and distribution of the drug.

Because of concern about the risks associated with the use of barbiturates, many physicians turned to other varieties of central nervous system depressants. However, these prescription sedatives, such as glutethimide (Doriden), ethchlorvynol (Placidyl), methaqualone (Quaalude), and methyprylon (Noludar), differ only slightly in pharmacological action from barbiturates, and most of the hazards of these drugs—including the possibility of addiction—are just about the same as for barbiturates.

In the case of flurazepam (Dalmane) and other benzodiazepines (Librium, Valium), there is less evidence that they are involved in "hard" addiction in the sense of "street abuse." But long-term use, which may be considered a form of dependence, is common with the benzodiazepines.

Dalmane, an effective sleep-inducer, is the only benzodiazepine marketed exclusively as a hypnotic, and it has cornered the market. The drug was originally touted as having no "hangover" effects, but disturbed coordination can occur for a day or so after taking a single dose. (Librium and Valium are prescribed mainly for daytime anxiety, although many users reportedly take them at bedtime as well.)

---

*The nonmedical use of barbiturates and of other psychoactive drugs is explored in another Consumers Union book, *Licit and Illicit Drugs: The Consumers Union Report on Narcotics, Stimulants, Depressants, Inhalants, Hallucinogens, and Marijuana—including Caffeine, Nicotine, and Alcohol* by Edward M. Brecher and the Editors of Consumer Reports, 1972.

According to a report entitled "Sleeping Pills, Insomnia, and Medical Practice," published in 1979 by the Institute of Medicine (IOM) of the National Academy of Sciences, most benzodiazepines have active metabolites (by-products) that remain in the body longer than most barbiturates. This was reported to be particularly true of Dalmane, whose major long-lived metabolite can accumulate in the body especially when the drug is taken night after night. In studies summarized in the IOM report, it was found: "By the second week of consecutive nightly usage of the 30 mg dose the active metabolite of flurazepam . . . had accumulated to a level 4 to 6 times greater than on the first morning after use." (When Dalmane use is stopped, however, the rebound or withdrawal insomnia phenomenon discussed earlier apparently is not experienced.) The report went on: "A few drinks of alcohol at any time during a 24 hour period after one week of consecutive nightly usage of flurazepam could produce a deleterious effect on coordination."

Dalmane is not unique in that respect: With virtually all hypnotics, mixing with alcohol or other depressant drugs creates a lethal risk. What may be even worse is that with some hypnotics—and Dalmane is among them—people may not realize their coordination is impaired and this can be particularly hazardous to themselves and others.

According to the IOM report, "Although it has been estimated that in a given year more than one percent of the adult population will use sleeping pills on consecutive nights for a period of more than two months, little research has been conducted concerning the efficacy of long-term use of hypnotic medication for sleep. Of drugs marketed in the United States, only flurazepam has been shown to affect sleep for as long as 28 days of continuous use, and then only in 10 insomniac subjects. Most other hypnotics that have been studied in the sleep laboratory appear to lose their sleep-promoting properties within three to 14 days of continuous use." A controlled study of hypnotics reported in 1974 in *The Journal of the American Medical Association* demonstrated the relative ineffectiveness of barbiturates and other central nervous system depressants when taken by insomniacs for longer than a two-week period.

"No hypnotic," the IOM report said, "has . . . ever been fully assessed with daytime measures of patients' mood, occupational performance, memory, cognition, psychomotor abilities and driving skills; nor has any evidence been presented demonstrating that chronic insomniacs are better off during the day as a consequence of having taken sleeping medication at night."

Actually, the amount of prescribed hypnotics has been declining, the IOM report said. "In 1971, 41.7 million prescriptions were written, 47 percent of which were for barbiturates. By contrast, in 1977 only 25.6 million prescriptions were written for hypnotics, a decrease of 39 percent; 17 percent of these were for barbiturates and 53 percent (13.6 million prescriptions) were for the single drug flurazepam." Whether the incidence of insomnia was also down or the use of prescription hypnotics has been replaced by other self-administered treatment, especially alcohol, was not reported.

Patients who are prescribed hypnotic drugs should expect their physicians to give them clear directions for use and specific warnings about possible side effects. In particular, patients should be aware of the following.

- Because flurazepam (Dalmane) lingers in the body and has a cumulative effect, patients should avoid driving (or operating machinery) at any time they feel even slightly drowsy. If they do expect to drive (or operate machinery), they should abstain from alcohol—day and night—while under treatment with the drug.

- Barbiturates may cause a "hangover" effect for the first few mornings after use is begun. What's more, use of barbiturates can interfere with anticoalgulant medications and may also alter the action of other drugs, both prescription and OTC. People who take barbiturates may need to consult their physician (or pharmacist) about possible interactions between barbiturates and other drugs.
- Pregnant women and women of child-bearing age who wish to become pregnant should not use hypnotics except under the close supervision of a physician.
- It is possible to develop dependence on hypnotics, if taken nightly.
- Alcohol, when used with any hypnotic, sedative, or tranquilizer, can be hazardous.

As for OTC "sleep aids," they are neither barbiturates nor tranquilizers. *Dormin, Nite Rest, Nytol,* and *Sominex,* like almost all other OTC sleeping preparations, contain an antihistamine as their main active ingredient. Until recently, methapyrilene was the antihistamine in most OTC sleep remedies. As noted in Chapter 1, in spring 1979 methapyrilene was found to be carcinogenic in laboratory animals and was considered to pose a potential risk to humans. Most OTC products containing the drug were recalled from the market. With the ban on methapyrilene, many sleep aids using that drug were reformulated with the antihistamine pyralimine. Another antihistamine, doxylamine succinate, is the active ingredient of a new product in the sleep-aid marketplace. Available OTC, *Unisom* is sold in dosages of 25 milligrams (mg). (Curiously, the same antihistamine, in 10 mg dosage, is found in the prescription drug Bendectin for the treatment of nausea and vomiting of pregnancy.)

Consumers Union's medical consultants question the use of antihistamines as sleep aids. Such products rely on a side effect

—drowsiness—and at the same time expose users to other possible side effects, such as dryness of the mouth, throat, and nose, nausea, vomiting, dizziness, frequent urination, fatigue, and double vision. Discomfort from use of antihistamines is far from uncommon. Goodman and Gilman, *The Pharmacological Basis of Therapeutics* notes: "About one person in four will experience some bothersome reaction during treatment with a given antihistamine."

Many people who complain about sleep problems actually sleep more than they think they do. Sleep disorder specialists estimate that one-third to one-half of all people who consider themselves insomniacs get as much sleep as people who consider themselves normal sleepers. When 122 insomniacs were studied in one sleep laboratory, most of them overestimated the time it took to fall asleep and underestimated their total sleep time.

If you are moved to "take something" for insomnia, a glass of warm milk at bedtime is certainly safer for most people than several drinks of alcohol, and recent research suggests that it just might work. Milk, meat, and a few other foods contain the amino acid L-tryptophan. Preliminary studies have shown that in mild insomniacs and in normal sleepers L-tryptophan taken as a drug reduces the time it takes to fall asleep and lengthens total sleep time. But more studies are necessary to establish its effectiveness and long-term safety.

Whether or not you take sleeping pills or other sleep aids, sleep specialists offer a number of general suggestions to help you fall asleep and sleep better.

- Avoid napping in the daytime and after dinner. Napping can cut down on sleep time at night.
- Don't drink beverages or take medications containing caffeine or use other stimulants (see page 284) for several hours prior to bedtime.

- Exercise frequently. Physical activity can be conducive to longer, deeper sleep. Sexual activity can also be an effective soporific for some people.
- Establish a regular schedule, including a time to go to bed and to wake up. Once the body is "programmed" for a daily sleep-wake cycle, sleep is easier to attain.
- Establish a regular bedtime ritual before retiring, such as taking a hot bath, reading, or anything else that's relaxing.
- If you're not sleepy, get out of bed. Pick up a book or turn on the radio or television. Soft music or a late night movie has restored many to peaceful slumber. Tossing and turning and worrying about falling asleep can only increase frustration. Remember that missing even an entire night or two of sleep has no known serious effects—except perhaps for the worry about not having slept.
- If the insomnia lasts for several weeks and doesn't respond to the above measures, consult a physician.

Until recently, OTC daytime sedatives were marketed to relieve "nervous tension," for "a relaxed feeling," or as something for "resolving that irritability that ruins your day." Most of these products contained antihistamines, thus counting on drowsiness—a known side effect—to make people feel less anxious. The FDA advisory panel reviewing OTC daytime sedative drug products could find no data "to indicate that the drowsiness effect is related to relieving symptoms of anxiety." As a result, based on the evidence, the FDA held that "no ingredient can be generally recognized as safe and effective for use as an OTC daytime sedative" and banned the sale of such products after December 24, 1979.

Another class of drugs, which is normally prescribed for tension or anxiety but is sometimes taken for insomnia, is the minor tranquilizers, such as meprobamate (Equanil, Miltown), chlordiazepoxide (Librium), diazepam (Valium), and others.

According to advertisements addressed to physicians in medical journals, these indeed must have been miracle drugs. One product, it was alleged, "helps restore the zest for living." Another was said to be useful "in emotional distress." A third "controls anxiety, tension, agitation, irritability, anxiety-linked depression," and so on. The ads urged physicians to prescribe one antianxiety drug for "emotional crises in office practice" and "to gain more immediate control of acute agitation and tension." Another drug was offered for the emotional aspects of physical illnesses—"when constant business worries aggravate peptic ulcer symptoms" or "when constant family pressures aggravate the symptoms of mild ulcerative colitis." Yet another drug was recommended "when your patient's worries, apprehensions, or other manifestations of acute and chronic anxiety interfere with his sleep"; then "a bedtime dosage . . . helps break the anxiety-insomnia cycle."

Such ads were for the most part based on the reports of physicians who had prescribed antianxiety drugs in their practice. Typical of such uncontrolled studies was one reported by a physician who prescribed diazepam (Valium) for seventy-four patients—men and women who came to him complaining of inability to sleep, "nervousness," tension, fatigue, crying spells, restlessness, and headache. The results seemed promising indeed. Of the seventy-four patients given diazepam, "improvement was marked in forty-five (60.8 percent), moderate in twenty (27 percent) and minimal in nine (12.2 percent)." Apparently, none failed to improve. Other uncontrolled studies of diazepam also brought glowing reports. One enthusiastic physician claimed that 58 to 93 percent of patients benefited.

In addition to anecdotal findings by physicians and their patients, there are reports of fully controlled clinical trials conducted by the Veterans Administration (VA) and the National

Institute of Mental Health (NIMH). In such trials, patients are placed at random into two groups. One group is given the test drug while the other is given a placebo, which looks like the study drug but contains no active ingredient. Such controlled trials are usually double-blind—neither the patients nor the physicians know which group has received the drug under investigation until the study is over and the results have been recorded. Also possible are crossover trials in which the patient receives the study drug for a period of time and then the placebo is given for a similar time span. Neither the patient nor the physician knows when the crossover takes place. In short, the test results are not biased by the patient's or the physician's thoughts about the medication. In many studies, objective tests are also given before and after drug or placebo treatment, and the drug is evaluated on the basis of comparative test scores.

When antianxiety drugs are tested in these sophisticated ways, a remarkable pattern is noted. In one controlled, double-blind study, for example, half of the patients given diazepam was judged to be significantly improved after six weeks on the basis of both objective tests and physician judgment. *But half of the patients given the placebo was also found to be significantly improved.*

With a few exceptions, the results of fully controlled trials using other leading antianxiety medications have been much the same. "Drugs such as meprobamate (Equanil or Miltown) and chlordiazepoxide (Librium) generally come out as being a little better than a placebo, but not by any dramatic margin," reported Jonathan O. Cole, M.D., formerly in charge of NIMH drug research studies and now chief of the psychopharmacology program at McLean Hospital, Belmont, Massachusetts. And, according to Goodman and Gilman, *The Pharmacological Basis of Therapeutics:* "The pharmacological effects of meprobamate are very similar to those of barbiturates. Indeed, in clinical usage it is difficult, if not impossible, to differentiate between the two drugs."

Not all authorities agreed with this view. "Our experiences in the VA would certainly give the antianxiety drugs higher marks than the barbiturates, both as to efficacy and safety," said Samuel C. Kaim, M.D., formerly in charge of research in psychiatry and neurology for the VA. "In several double-blind studies, meprobamate and chlordiazepoxide have turned out to be better than either barbiturates or a placebo." This view is shared by the countless physicians who prescribe antianxiety drugs, and of the patients who report benefits from them. Although no final resolution of this controversy is in sight, *AMA Drug Evaluations* commented that antianxiety agents "may be useful for patients in whom the sedative-hypnotics cause an excessive loss of alertness."

Cole called attention to an unusual finding: "In a series of studies involving three out-patient clinics," he noted, "we have been most struck by the fact that the results differ substantially from clinic to clinic, to the extent that if each clinic were considered as a single study, quite different results would have been reported. . . . These differences cannot be accounted for by the known characteristics of the patients treated."

To sum up the evidence on effectiveness, the odds are slightly better than fifty-fifty that a patient given an antianxiety drug by a physician will be benefited. Patients in need of sedation are the ones most likely to benefit. If the physician has faith in the drug, the results are likely to be good. These findings explain why antianxiety drugs are so popular. Whether they work more frequently than a placebo or not, whether they work differently from a barbiturate or not—they do relieve the symptoms of anxiety in a significant percentage of cases.

There is little to guide a physician in selecting one antianxiety drug over another. There have been few well-controlled comparison trials on these drugs, and "clinical experience does not clearly point to any one of them as outstanding," *The Medical Letter* has noted. "In the absence of a sound basis for a choice, picking a drug for a patient hampered by anxiety must be more or less arbitrary; if one is not effective, or causes unwanted side effects, another can be tried."

The Pharmacological Basis of Therapeutics points to the inherent difficulties of diagnosing anxiety and of deciding how it might be treated. It goes on to state that "the *selection* of an antianxiety drug is less of a problem than the initial decision to use one." Among possible treatments suggested in Goodman and Gilman are an alcoholic beverage, for some older people; long-acting barbiturates (such as phenobarbital), which are inexpensive and well tolerated; and benzodiazepines (such as chlordiazepoxide or diazepam).

There are potential side effects and, indeed, dangers associated with drugs used for anxiety. Among the side effects reported for the minor tranquilizers are drowsiness—the most common—and an occasional stomach upset. Allergic reactions, usually consisting of a skin rash, may develop. Bone marrow changes, which normally are reversible when the drug is discontinued, occasionally occur. "In general," the *VA Bulletin* noted, "the disturbances are neither severe nor especially common." Minor side effects appear—and usually soon disappear —early in the course of treatment.

Drowsiness is a real hazard in patients who drive a car or operate some type of machinery. Lack of coordination can also be a problem. *Patients on minor tranquilizers should not drink alcoholic beverages, or take antihistamines or sedatives.* Tranquilizers, sedatives, antihistamines, and alcohol all tend to slow reaction time, interfere with coordination, and cause drowsiness. The effects of alcohol consumption alone on traffic accident rates have long been known. Some observers now see a relationship between widespread use of minor tranquilizers—with or without alcohol—and high accident rates. Such effects can be dangerously exaggerated when two or more of these drugs are taken together; and driving becomes even more of a hazard. As with anti-insomnia medication, daytime drowsiness and decreased coordination is also possible after nighttime use of antianxiety medication. Such effects, of course, are also possible with the frequent use of alcohol in large dosages as self-treatment for anxiety.

In 1978 the FDA ordered manufacturers of antianxiety prescription drugs to change their labeling to state that the drugs have not been demonstrated effective when taken by patients consistently for extended periods.

The following statement has been added to the labeling of all antianxiety drugs: "The effectiveness of [drug name] in long term use, that is, more than 4 months, has not been assessed by systematic clinical studies. The physician should periodically reassess the usefulness of the drug for the individual patient."

The requirement grew out of a recommendation made by the FDA's Psychopharmacological Agents Advisory Committee. The committee said that the long-term use of antianxiety drugs—in the absence of other measures designed to combat or alter the situation causing the distress or the individual's response to it—is unwise. (According to CU's medical consultants, the same can be said for long-term use of alcohol.)

As *The Pharmacological Basis of Therapeutics* puts it, "Long courses of treatment are rarely needed or useful since tolerance develops to [central nervous system] depressants and anxiety is usually self-limited. Prolonged therapy can lead to habituation and little therapeutic effect. . . ."

25

Buying
prescription drugs

Prescription drug sales in the United States came to about $13 billion in 1978. Profits enjoyed by drug manufacturers have been equally impressive. Over the past decade or so the drug industry has ranked among the top two or three most profitable manufacturing industries in the country.

For many years Consumers Union has tried to help consumers avoid contributing unduly to the high profits of drug companies. CU has advised those who purchase prescription drugs —especially the higher-priced ones—to try to save money by buying, whenever possible, the generic form of the drug, which may cost less than the brand-name version of the product. Since prices vary from pharmacy to pharmacy, CU has also urged consumers who are not confronted with a medical emergency to take the time to comparison shop before having a prescription filled.

Indeed, numerous surveys have repeatedly documented the wide disparity in pricing of prescription drugs—and the value of comparison shopping. For example, CU made a prescription shopping test in the New York metropolitan area some time ago. Given a prescription for thirty capsules of tetracycline, the generic name for a commonly used broad-spectrum antibiotic (see Chapter 26), CU shoppers went to sixty drugstores. The prices they had to pay ranged from 79 cents all the way to $7.45. The results of CU's test shopping have been confirmed by other agencies—governmental, trade, and private—that have undertaken similar drug price surveys.

The American Medical Association (AMA) made a study a while back in the Chicago area. AMA shoppers filled 686 prescriptions for seven drugs at 185 drugstores. One of the drugs bought was meprobamate, marketed as Miltown by Wallace, as Equanil by Wyeth, and by generic name by other companies. In all, 159 prescriptions for this drug were filled, each calling for twenty-five tablets containing 0.4 grams per tablet. Forty-nine pharmacies filled prescriptions calling for Miltown at prices ranging from $1.63 to $4.95. Sixty-two prescriptions calling for the same amount of Equanil were filled at prices ranging from $1.72 to $4.05. Prescriptions calling only for meprobamate, without specifying a brand name, were filled by forty-eight pharmacies. Half of them supplied either Miltown or Equanil, at prices ranging from $1.25 to $4.40. The other half provided tablets not identifiable by brand name, at prices ranging from $1.25 to $4.00. (Startling variations were also found in the prices charged for the other drugs in the AMA survey.)

According to the Department of Health, Education, and Welfare (HEW), 90 percent of all prescriptions written in the United States are for brand-name drugs and some of those drugs cost up to seven times the cost of their generic equivalent. In an attempt to encourage increased use of cheaper generic drugs, HEW has provided states with a model generic drug law and issued a list of generic drugs that are the therapeutic equivalent of name brands. Forty-six states have some type of generic drug law (see page 306).

Until recent years, few consumers had easy access to price

information about prescription drugs. The laws and regulations of many states prohibited the advertising of prescription drug prices. In other states pharmaceutical trade groups and state boards of pharmacy tended to pressure stores not to post prices or advertise prescription costs. To some extent, these practices were challenged in court cases that upheld the right of several large drug chains to make price information public. Accelerating the process of informing the public were federal anti-inflation measures in 1972, which required pharmacies to compile data about pricing and to make the information available to customers who requested it.

Several states ultimately forced the issue. New York State pharmacists have been required since January 1, 1974, to post prominently the names and prices of the 150 most frequently prescribed drugs. (Boston has enforced such regulations since 1971.) As of late 1979, Arkansas, California, Connecticut, Louisiana, Maine, Maryland, Michigan, Minnesota, Nevada, New Hampshire, Rhode Island, South Dakota, Texas, Washington, West Virginia, and Washington, D.C., also require posting some prescription drug prices.

The Food and Drug Administration (FDA) intervened toward the close of 1973 to help standardize the pricing information to be given to consumers. Since January 1976, the agency has prescribed the format to be used for posting and advertising of prescription drug prices. Through its regulations, the FDA hopes to ensure a uniform national system that will provide consumers "with information needed to make meaningful price comparisons."

CU reminds consumers that until states require pharmacies to post the prices of *all* drugs, it may pay to check on the cost of a prescription before it is filled, and then compare the price at another pharmacy.

Even if all states were to require full disclosure of prescription drug prices, there would still be limits to the efficacy of comparison shopping for drugs. Because of the nature of the drug industry, and the effect of patent laws, certain drugs dominate the United States market. And in some instances, the cooperation of your physician and pharmacist will be necessary. The following review of the process by which new prescription drugs are marketed may, to some extent, help consumers avoid overspending for medications.

During the period in which a new drug is undergoing clinical investigation, it is given its *generic* name by the United States Adopted Names Council (a semiofficial organization sponsored by the AMA, the United States Pharmacopeial Convention, and the American Pharmaceutical Association). The generic name is usually a simplified word version of the chemical formulation. Once the FDA has declared the drug to be both safe and effective, and therefore ready for marketing, the pharmaceutical firm decides on a *brand* name for its new product; this name is then registered as a trademark. From the manufacturer's point of view, the ideal brand name is one that will stick tenaciously in the memory of prescribing physicians.

Patent rights, ordinarily lasting for seventeen years, protect the new drug from duplication by rival firms. During that period, the company holding the patent enjoys exclusive rights to production and sales—unless it decides to license, for a fee, other firms to market the drug. If the patent holder decides not to license another manufacturer, a prescription written for the new drug by its generic name will cost as much as one written by its brand name during the life of the patent. For example, diazepam—better known by its brand name, Valium—was developed by Hoffmann-La Roche, the world's largest drug company. With other firms excluded from production while the patent is in effect, prescriptions written for diazepam could be filled only with Valium.

When a patent expires, other firms may then manufacture the drug. The original patent holder, however, retains the right to the brand name. Competing companies must market the product under its generic name or invent their own brand names. So-called branded generics, which have been developed by some of the larger pharmaceutical houses, sell at a competitive price but retain some brand-name characteristics. One example is Robitet, A. H. Robins's branded-generic version of tetracycline, which sells for less than Achromycin, the brand-name tetracycline marketed by Lederle, the original patent holder.

Once the patent expires, the price of the original brand-name drug may fall. The cut in price is affected by the number of competing products, market demand, and promotion to physicians. Despite advertising to physicians and efforts of rival detail men and women (see Chapter 27), the original drug firm retains a considerable advantage even after the patent rights expire, because the medical profession has for so long equated the product with the original brand name. Eli Lilly & Co. still enjoys large profits from the sale of Darvon (a prescription analgesic with the generic name propoxyphene), despite the expiration of patent rights, and despite the fact that smaller companies sell their versions of propoxyphene for a fraction of the price charged for Darvon. Doctors who specify a brand name in a prescription in effect compel their patients to enrich the manufacturer of that brand-name drug.

Brand-name prescription drugs often cost five to ten times more than their generic counterparts—and sometimes even up to thirty times more. Understandably, the drug industry has not been enthusiastic about the efforts of CU and other consumer organizations and of legislators who advocate prescription by generic name. Industry representatives often question the quality of generic drugs. CU's medical consultants believe that the price of a medicine is not necessarily a reliable guide to its quality.

The quality of prescription drugs marketed in the United States is monitored by the FDA through large centers for drug analysis. The National Center for Antibiotics in Washington, D.C., is responsible for certifying the potency, purity, and stability of every antibiotic, batch by batch, prior to marketing. Of the other drug-testing centers, for example, the National Center for Drug Analysis in St. Louis has since 1970 completed studies of thirty-four classes of drugs, including, among others, adrenocorticosteroids, major and minor tranquilizers, urinary antibacterial agents, central nervous system depressants, antithyroid agents, cardiac drugs, anticoagulants, and oral contraceptives. The survey covers every known manufacturer of the most important drug classes.

Such efforts on the part of the FDA led Henry E. Simmons, M.D., then head of its Bureau of Drugs, to state in 1972: "On the basis of the data we have accrued to date we cannot conclude there is a significant difference in quality between the generic and brand-name product tested." Both large and small pharmaceutical firms have had quality control problems.

In 1978 in testimony before the House Subcommittee on Consumer Protection and Finance, Donald Kennedy, Ph.D., then FDA commissioner, affirmed the FDA's view that there is no widespread difference in quality among drugs approved by the FDA, whether they are sold under a generic name or under a heavily advertised brand name.

Proponents of brand-name drugs have questioned not only the quality but also therapeutic equivalence of brand-name and generic products. An important factor in the determination of therapeutic equivalence is the bioavailability of a drug. In the case of a drug taken orally, this represents the amount of active medication absorbed from the intestine into the bloodstream, thus making the drug available to perform its biological function. Bioavailability can be evaluated by analyzing the blood of patients who have ingested a drug. In such fashion, blood levels of chemically identical drugs can be compared and, if found similar, therapeutic equivalence may be presumed. Differences in bioavailability have been attributed to variations in the formulation of products. Drug companies may use a variety of inert ingredients, known to the trade as stabilizers, binders, and so forth, in the manufacturing process. These ingredients may or may not affect absorption of a drug (and thus its bioavailability).

The United States Pharmacopeia (USP) sets the standards for laboratory testing of drugs to ensure quality and purity. One test related to the question of bioavailability is that for dissolution—how quickly the active ingredient in, say, a tablet being tested passes into solution. In contrast to tests for disintegration—how quickly the tablet breaks up into smaller particles of specified size—performance in dissolution tests does correlate with bioavailability. Beginning in 1970, dissolution time specifications have been required by the USP for several drug classes including digoxin (a commonly used heart drug), hydrochlorothiazide (a diuretic), phenylbutazone (an anti-inflammatory drug), prednisone (a cortisone analogue), sulfisoxazole and nitrofurantoin (urinary antibiotics), and tolbutamide (an oral hypoglycemic). CU's medical consultants endorse the addition of dissolution time tests to USP standards for these drugs and applaud the fact that the USP's goal is now to include the information for virtually all drugs. The tightening of standards helps ensure the therapeutic equivalence of chemically identical drugs made by different manufacturers, as well as different batches of a drug made by the same firm. With more drugs on the list, the chances of differences in bioavailability will be narrowed even further.

The actual number of instances in which differences in bioavailability have been demonstrated are relatively small—a fraction of the prescription drug market. With the current FDA and USP controls in operation, defective products and differences in bioavailability are less likely to go undetected.

The generic versus brand name controversy is part of a long struggle between consumer groups and the drug industry to lower drug costs without sacrificing quality. CU believes that the use of brand names for drugs should be completely eliminated, and that all drugs should be designated only by generic name. If the belief persists that price is indicative of quality—or if the last sales pitch casts a spell—a physician could still specify a particular manufacturer's more costly version. But when no manufacturer is singled out on the prescription blank, the mandatory use of the generic name should help the consumer to purchase the least expensive alternative, should there be several equivalent products on the pharmacist's shelves.

In 1978 nearly a dozen prescriptions were written for each American, on average. Prescription drugs accounted for about $70 of the $737 per capita costs of health care. However, the price of drugs is not shared equally across the boards: The elderly and the chronically ill have the greatest need for drugs and—in general—they have the lowest income.

In addition to savings for the consumer, the elimination of brand names for prescription drugs might also benefit some doctors—and ultimately their patients. The FDA has estimated that about 700 prescription drugs are marketed under about 20,000 brand names—which means an average of about twenty-eight different names for each prescription drug. The profusion of brand names inevitably creates confusion for many busy physicians. The tale has been told of a hapless physician who prescribed Lederle's Achromycin for a patient's respiratory infection. When the patient showed no improvement, the doctor then prescribed, also to no avail, Squibb's Sumycin, followed by Bristol's Tetrex, little realizing that these were all brand names for the same drug, tetracycline. If CU's proposal for the mandatory use of generic names were fully implemented, there would be less reason to repeat such stories.

Physicians have had increased incentive to prescribe generically as a result of a program announced by the secretary of HEW in December 1973. At that time, the secretary said that the department proposed to limit reimbursement for any drug under Medicare and Medicaid "to the lowest cost at which the drug is generally available unless there is a demonstrated difference in therapeutic effect." Operative since August 1976, the Maximum Allowable Cost program began slowly but is now, according to HEW, "a very effective cost containment project."

Even with the exclusive use of generic names for prescription drugs, much would still depend on the pharmacist, as well as on the commitment of the consumer to comparison shopping. For example, there are no cost benefits for the patient who brings a prescription for generic ampicillin (an antibiotic) to a pharmacist who stocks only Bristol's brand, Polycillin. The pharmacist may legally sell a higher-priced brand-name product if a generic is specified. Therefore, a consumer whose physician has written a generic prescription must still check prices at a few pharmacies in order to obtain the lowest price. In four states—Hawaii, Indiana, Mississippi, and Texas—pharmacists are forbidden to substitute a generic drug for a prescribed brand name.

In New York State, a physician's prescription form must carry by law the following: "Dispense as written" or "Substitution permissible." The physician issuing the prescription will sign one or the other. Under the physician's signature is the sentence: "This prescription will be filled generically unless physician signs the line stating 'dispense as written.' "

Here are some additional suggestions about prescription drugs from CU's medical consultants.

- Discuss with your physician the side effects, the correct dosage, and time for taking a prescribed drug. Ask that the prescription state that these medication instructions be included on the drug label. Advice to "Take as directed" is not much help if you forget the doctor's instructions—or never clearly understood them in the first place.

- For drugs that are taken regularly, check to see if you can save money by buying as large a quantity as will stay fresh at the rate you use them (ask your pharmacist).

- If your state does not now have such a requirement, ask your physician to direct the pharmacist to include on each prescription drug label the name of the drug, its strength, the amount (number of tablets, ounces, etc.), and the expiration date (the date after which the medication is no longer sure to be fully effective, or may be harmful). With this information available to you, leftover portions of some prescriptions could still be used if the physician should prescribe the same medication again. Do not, however, use such leftovers until you have checked with your doctor and confirmed that they are the correct medicine in the proper dosage. Such information on the label also could be life-saving should anyone take an overdose of a medication.

- Make sure you keep your physician informed of all the drugs you normally take—both prescription and over the counter. Such information may help to prevent adverse drug interactions.

- Discard all prescription drugs by their expiration date.

- If you find child-resistant medicine containers difficult to open—and there are no young children in your household

—ask the pharmacist to put your medication in an ordinary container.

- Some consumers may have no choice about where to fill a prescription—especially in an emergency situation. Even for those who can shop around, it may be best to stick with a single pharmacy once comparison pricing has shown the charges to be consistently reasonable. The price differential between a neighborhood drugstore and a pharmacy in a large cut-rate drugstore or in a department store may be less important than the service extras the local pharmacy may offer. The neighborhood pharmacist usually keeps records of your purchases of prescription medications. Such records can be important in preventing or tracing allergic reactions to drugs; they also can help avoid the dispensing of incompatible drugs. For those who can afford the markup, such personal service, plus home delivery (if available), and possible assistance in emergencies, may be worth the extra money involved.

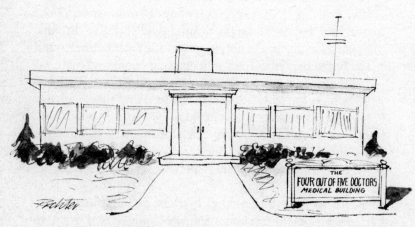

Drawing by Richter; © 1979 The New Yorker Magazine, Inc.

26
The other side
of antibiotics

Antibiotics have eliminated or controlled so many infectious diseases that almost everyone has benefited from their use at one time or another. Even without such personal experience, however, one would have to be isolated indeed to be unaware of the virtues—real and alleged—of these drugs. Their truly remarkable success in the chemical war on bacteria has been extensively reported by the press, television, and radio. And any gap in the media accounts has been more than compensated for by the aggressive public relations activity of the pharmaceutical manufacturers who sell antibiotics.

In contrast, the inadequacies and potential dangers of these remarkable drugs are much less widely known. The lack of such knowledge often leads patients to pressure their doctors into prescribing antibiotics for illnesses that cannot be benefited by such therapy. Unfortunately, an alarming number of physicians are willing to comply with patients' demands for antibiotics. One study completed several years ago showed that 90 percent of penicillin usage was inappropriate. It has been estimated that 50 percent of all patients who see their doctor for the common cold receive an antibiotic. Since this is a viral illness the drug is useless. Surveys of the use of antibiotics in hospitals reveal that 60 percent of the patients receive either an incorrect antibiotic, or the wrong dosage, or a drug when none is required.

Because the positive side of the antibiotics story is so well known, it seems more useful here to review some of the immediate and long-range problems that can result from indiscriminate use of these drugs. It should be understood that calamities from the use of antibiotics are rare in proportion to the enormous amounts of these potent drugs being administered to patients. But the potential hazards, so little touched on generally, need greater emphasis.

Almost all antibiotics are prescription drugs. A few antibiotics, however, are permitted in such over-the-counter (OTC) products as nasal sprays, lozenges, troches, creams, and ointments. Even if these products do no harm—a claim that can be questioned, especially in regard to the development of resistant bacteria (discussed below)—there is little benefit in using them. If you have an infection serious enough to warrant the launching of chemical warfare, you need antibiotics in a form and dosage prescribed by a physician, not in nonprescription products for self-medication. What's more, even small amounts of an OTC antibiotic ointment can cause an allergic skin reaction.

Antibiotics are far from being a sure cure-all. There are wide gaps in their ability to master infectious diseases. Such important viral infections as the common cold and infectious hepatitis still await conquest. A good deal of progress has been made in the chemotherapy of some viral illnesses, but more investigation is needed before these agents are perfected.

The numerous bacteria that cause infectious diseases can be identified in the laboratory by the way the bacteria grow on certain culture media and by a color reaction that takes place on a glass slide when the bacteria are stained with certain chemicals. This is known as the Gram's stain technique. When the slide is viewed under a microscope some bacteria are stained blue (Gram-positive) while the others are stained red (Gram-negative).

Antibiotics such as clindamycin, erythromycin, penicillin, and vancomycin act on Gram-positive organisms and are considered narrow-spectrum agents. Ampicillin, the cephalosporins, chloramphenicol, gentamicin, and tetracycline act on both Gram-positive and Gram-negative organisms. These are considered broad-spectrum antibiotics. In general, the most specific agent should be used for the bacteria causing the illness. When initiating therapy for a serious infection, one or two broad-spectrum agents are often utilized pending the isolation of the particular bacteria involved.

Antibiotics can be classified also as bacteriostatic or bactericidal. Bacteriostatic antibiotics, such as tetracycline, prevent multiplication of the bacterial population and allow natural body mechanisms to take over and heal the infection. Bactericidal antibiotics, such as penicillin, actually destroy the organism. When an exact diagnosis has been made, and the choice of antibiotics is between one that is bacteriostatic or one that is bactericidal, the latter is usually preferred.

In time, certain bacteria become resistant to antibiotics. Because of the widespread use of antibiotics that destroy Gram-positive bacteria, Gram-negative types are assuming increasing clinical importance. At least one researcher has estimated that Gram-negative bacteria cause serious blood serum infections in about 1 percent of patients in hospitals and result in the death of about 100,000 Americans each year.

It has been well established that the increase in strains of bacteria resistant to a particular antibiotic correlates directly with inadequate dosage and inappropriate use. For example, one hospital survey showed that before erythromycin was widely used there, all strains of staphylococci found in patients and staff personnel were sensitive to this antibiotic's action. When doctors at the hospital started extensive use of erythromycin, however, resistant staphylococcal strains began to appear.

The development of bacterial resistance can be minimized by more discriminating use of antibiotics. When an antibiotic must be used, the best way to prevent the development of resistance is to wipe out the infection rapidly and thoroughly. It is of utmost importance that adequate dosage be taken by patients. The doctor selects the drug, but patients must be responsible for completing the full course of the recommended treatment, even though the symptoms may disappear before the prescribed amount of medication has been taken. In many instances patients will initiate therapy on their own with antibiotics that have been left over from a previous illness or that have been prescribed for another member of the family. In addition to being potentially dangerous, indiscriminate use of an antibiotic may make diagnosis and proper treatment of a serious illness more difficult.

As with other drugs, antibiotics may sensitize a patient so that subsequent use of that medication will induce an allergic reaction. This reaction can vary from a mild skin rash to an immediate life-threatening situation called anaphylactic shock. Up to 5 percent of patients receiving penicillin will experience an allergic reaction. Fortunately, only 1 in 100,000 patients will develop anaphylaxis. Anaphylactic shock can also be caused by bee stings (see page 173). Indeed, on rare occasions, it may follow an injection of virtually any substance. Within minutes after taking the offending medication—usually a penicillin injection—the patient begins to experience difficulty in breathing, accompanied by a tight feeling in the chest and possibly by severe generalized itching. Collapse and death may follow;

life-saving treatment consists of an immediate injection of adrenaline followed by an antihistamine. Consumers Union's medical consultants urge all patients to wait at least ten minutes in the doctor's office or clinic after receiving an injection of penicillin to make sure that if anaphylactic shock does occur, immediate treatment is available.

Anaphylactic shock usually happens without warning, often in a patient with no history of penicillin allergy. Fortunately, as pointed out, anaphylactic shock is uncommon. The more typical allergic reaction to penicillin takes the form of a generalized itchy rash or hives, which usually develops during the time the medication is being taken or up to two weeks following discontinuance. The rash may persist from several days to a week or more and may cause severe discomfort. The allergic reaction itself is best treated by an antihistamine; in severe cases, corticosteroids may be necessary. Itching may be helped by the use of analgesics, such as aspirin or acetaminophen, as well as by cool cornstarch baths.

It is unlikely that someone using a drug for the very first time will develop an allergic reaction to it. However, the initial contact with the sensitizing drug may have been inadvertent. For example, many years ago penicillin was used by the brewing industry to prevent bacterial contamination in the fermenting process. And some beer drinkers may have received a small sensitizing dose of penicillin along with their brew. Thus some subsequent exposure to penicillin—say, as medication—could precipitate an allergic reaction in sensitized beer drinkers.

The interval between the time of initial exposure and the first allergic reaction may be as short as a few days or may extend over several years. For reasons that are as yet unclear, an individual can become sensitized and have an allergic reaction to a medication even after taking the drug uneventfully many times. Once an allergy to a medication has been well documented, it would seem prudent to avoid that medication even to the extent of carrying a wallet card alerting others to that fact. Also possible is an allergic reaction to an antibiotic similar in chemical structure to one that is a known allergen for that patient. Thus a patient who is sensitive to penicillin may show an allergic reaction to cephalosporin.

To minimize the risk of anaphylactic shock in illnesses in which penicillin is the preferred treatment, a doctor questions the patient carefully about previous allergic reactions to drugs. In case of doubt, another antibiotic may be substituted. Although attempting to avoid a reaction is important, it is also necessary, especially in the treatment of serious diseases, not to restrict the use of an indicated drug, such as penicillin, because of a vague history of "allergy." Many so-called allergic reactions are, in fact, side effects of antibiotic use, such as stomach upset or diarrhea.

Some side effects of antibiotics may indeed be troublesome. A sore mouth, a "furry" tongue, cramps, diarrhea, anal itch, vaginal itch, nausea, vomiting, and so on, occur most frequently after oral use of a broad-spectrum antibiotic, most commonly tetracycline. (For the reason why tetracycline should not be taken toward the end of pregnancy, see page 248.) These complications, which are not true allergic reactions, may result from direct irritative effects of the antibiotic on the stomach and the intestines, or from elimination by the antibiotic of harmless bacteria normally found in the gastrointestinal tract. With the natural balance of power destroyed, antibiotic-resistant staphylococci and fungi, which are normally present, are free to flourish and cause what is called a superinfection. Such infections can be quite debilitating and difficult to cure.

In women taking a broad-spectrum antibiotic, growth of the yeast monilia can cause a distressing vaginal itch and discharge for which treatment may be difficult. If a vaginal infection by monilia should develop during treatment with an antibiotic, it is best, in the opinion of CU's medical consultants, to treat the vaginal itch with adequate amounts of an antifungal agent such as nystatin (Mycostatin) in the form of intravaginal inserts.

A few antibiotics have such toxic side effects that their usefulness is strictly limited. They include such potent agents as amikacin and gentamicin, which can sometimes cause deafness as well as impairment of kidney function.

The story of chloramphenicol has been told in the pages of *Consumer Reports*—see, for example, the issue of October 1970. As Chloromycetin (its Parke, Davis trade name), this drug enjoyed great popularity in the 1950s. Its indiscriminate use for minor infections resulted in several well-publicized fatalities due to aplastic anemia, a disease of the bone marrow in which blood-forming elements are suppressed. The incidence of fatal bone marrow suppression due to chloramphenicol is rare. It occurs once in approximately 40,000 to 80,000 courses of therapy. As with most other medications, a benefit-to-risk ratio may indicate that this potent antibiotic be used in certain infections that are life threatening. In such situations, the drug is virtually always used intravenously. Chloramphenicol is the drug of choice for some infections of the brain and spinal cord membranes, Rocky Mountain spotted fever, and typhoid fever. It is also used in certain abdominal infections such as peritonitis.

One kind of aplastic anemia resulting from the use of chloramphenicol is irreversible and inevitably fatal. This hypersensitivity reaction of the bone marrow to chloramphenicol is not related to the amount of the drug taken and may follow the administration of even very small quantities. Fortunately, this phenomenon is very rare. The more common type of aplastic anemia following use of chloramphenicol *is* dose-related, and therefore is usually reversible once the drug has been discontinued. However, it is impossible to predict which type of aplastic anemia could occur in an individual who takes chloramphenicol. If used judiciously for appropriate causes, there is no doubt that chloramphenicol is a valuable drug. Since patients with diseases serious enough to warrant consideration of this agent are usually hospitalized, some authorities have sought to restrict the drug to in-hospital use only. CU's medical consultants agree: Chloramphenicol should have no place in routine outpatient office practice.

The selection of the appropriate antibiotic usually takes a little time. A physician's selection may be influenced by testing the infecting organism for its susceptibility to various antibiotics. It is usually possible to detect the infecting organism by means of a bacteriological smear and culture. In the case of a respiratory infection or pneumonia, this may be done by a throat or sputum culture. Similarly, infected wounds, urine, and stools may be cultured. When, in the course of a day or two, growth of the organism is noted on the culture medium, its susceptibility to various antibiotics may be tested and reported in order of effectiveness. The doctor then chooses the most effective antibiotic with the least side effects.

Another factor that might influence the physician's choice of an antibiotic is the site of the infection. For example, for an infection in the urinary tract the physician may prescribe an antibiotic that is excreted in high amounts in the urine. In some instances, the cost of a particular antibiotic might be the determining factor when a choice exists among several drugs with near-equal efficacy. And the cost to the patient of various antibiotics may often be less if the physician prescribes a drug by its generic name rather than by its brand name.

The expense and the possible troubles that can result from antibiotic treatment should not keep anyone from using one of these drugs when it is clearly necessary to do so. Nor should the possibility of such problems discourage certain preventive uses of antibiotics, which have proved extremely valuable.

There are relatively few occasions that call for the use of an antibiotic as a prophylactic medication, that is, to prevent an illness instead of to treat an illness. More often than not, antibiotics are misused when taken prophylactically. The most common misuse is their administration in the course of a common cold in order to prevent a secondary infection. Colds are self-limited viral infections that rarely develop complications. Antibiotics for the common cold are an unnecessary expense and put the patient at risk for a possible drug reaction.

In patients with known rheumatic heart disease, implanted artificial heart valves, and other heart valve disorders, however, antibiotics *should* be used prophylactically prior to, during, and after dental extractions, drilling of cavities, and operations on the gastrointestinal or genitourinary tract. Such antibiotic prophylaxis can prevent subacute bacterial endocarditis (infection of a heart valve), a disease that is always serious and sometimes fatal.

In addition, young patients who have had one or more attacks of rheumatic fever may be able to avoid recurrences—which could result in new or further heart damage—with daily prophylactic doses of penicillin, continued well into adult life. (Erythromycin is a reasonable alternative in cases of penicillin allergy.) New cases of rheumatic fever are now uncommon, no doubt as a result of prompt recognition and treatment of streptococcal sore throats, which bear a causal relationship to acute rheumatic fever. Treatment of such sore throats usually consists of a ten-day course of penicillin.

People whose sexual partners are being treated for either gonorrhea or syphilis should consult a physician or a clinic for simultaneous treatment with an appropriate antibiotic, even if no symptoms are present. Antibiotics are used prophylactically for the immediate family of anyone diagnosed as having meningococcal meningitis.

Many surgeons feel that the prophylactic use of antibiotics can reduce the postoperative infection rate in most cases of cardiovascular, intestinal, and orthopedic (total hip replacement) surgery. If antibiotics are used as prophylaxes, they are usually given just prior to the operation and for less than twenty-four hours afterwards. Prolonged postoperative use of antibiotics has no added benefits and may have drawbacks.

The medical community has been made increasingly aware of the drawbacks and dangers—as well as the unnecessary expense—inherent in the overuse and misuse of antibiotic therapy. In many hospitals the newer, more potent antibiotics are restricted for use in specific clinical situations. All hospitals are now required to audit their use of antibiotics. It is hoped that the information gained from such reviews will lead to the more rational use of these important agents.

27

Evaluating news about miracles

In addition to the constant barrage of drug advertising, which some people have learned to disregard, drug publicity posing as news sends out subtler signals. Hardly a magazine appears on the stands without one or more medical articles; newspapers run medical columns and medical news; there is a steady outpouring of medical books for lay readers; and television and radio convey medical information not only in news and documentary programs but in hospital dramas and soap operas.

Some of this material is more or less accurate and helpful; a great deal of it is not. Much of what we read, see, and hear about medicine is inspired (and sometimes subsidized) by the publicity staffs of drug companies.

Drug publicity may go out under the firm's name, or it may issue from a "medical information bureau," a "medical news service," or some similar cover name designed to impress readers, writers, broadcast producers, and editors—and, possibly, to camouflage the backing of drug manufacturers. The objective is to get news of the product into newspapers and magazines and on radio and television. The theory—and it apparently works—is that if people learn about new drugs they will rush to their doctors' offices and demand them. Newspapers often publish promotion releases without distinguishing between what is scientifically valuable and what is pure promotional puffery. In magazines, a story may be signed by a free-lance or staff writer, but it is often inspired by a drug manufacturer's publicity bureau that has steered the writer to a researcher doing work for the company on one of its products. Some companies even subsidize the writing of free-lance articles later sold to magazines. The claims made in these articles often bear little or no relation to actual performance; indeed, some overly optimistic articles are based largely on what investigators *hope* they will find in research just getting under way.

The family doctor, who should be in a position to help patients appraise the optimistic press reports, barely has time to keep abreast of the steady flow of literature appearing in legitimate medical journals—let alone quasi-medical articles in the popular press. Even for a physician who keeps up with medical news, there are detail men and women to contend with —salespeople hired by drug companies to promote the companies' products. Most of the large companies employ hundreds of them, and they subject doctors to heavy sales pressure. The Council on Economic Priorities reports that in 1972 drug companies spent about $1 billion on promotion—the equivalent of $5,000 per doctor. And detail men and women represent about 70 percent of the promotional budget.

Under regulations of the Food and Drug Administration (FDA) manufacturers may not issue promotional material representing that a drug is safe or effective before the drug has been approved by the FDA. However, news reports may be circulated during the trial period, and it is entirely possible that such reports are partisan and misleading, even if they are not untrue.

Much pharmaceutical research is simply the offspring of competitive pressure. Many "new" products come out each year without regard to specific need for them in medical practice; only a few can be considered real advances in therapy. Most new products are in direct competition with older drugs made by other pharmaceutical companies. Sometimes a new drug is actually the same old drug, only with new use indications. Or established medications are sometimes combined, and the combination advertised to physicians as "new." Variations in the chemical formula of an old medication occasionally bring real improvement in a drug's action, or tone down some serious side effect. More often, a new formulation has little additional value except to the company holding the patent.

Many of the new forms and chemical variations go through a series of "research" stages; at each stage encouraging results are likely to be reported in the general press as well as in professional journals. In fact, most of these news stories herald a business coup, on a par with a paint company's discovery of a way to obtain a new shade of blue. Occasionally, a story may be planted at a strategic time to enhance the stock of a drug manufacturer.

The FDA has established a formal in-house system of classifications for new drugs. Its ratings are determined by the FDA's Bureau of Drugs, the section of the agency that assesses most new drug products submitted for marketing. The FDA ratings are based on staff scientists' evaluations of research data that the drug manufacturer must provide. Every drug approved by the Bureau of Drugs is rated with a number-letter classification that tells at a glance whether it is considered a medical breakthrough, a more modest advance, or offers little or no new benefit compared with existing drugs of its type.

Each rating includes two essential judgments. The first is conveyed by a number from 1 to 6 that indicates the drug's newness and uniqueness. The lower the number, the more novel the drug. The number 1, for example, is reserved for new molecular entities being marketed for the first time in the United States, while 5 means the product is an exact duplicate of a drug already manufactured by another firm—a "me-too drug," as it is called in the trade.

Each product's number designation is followed by a letter— usually A, B, or C. An A is "a breakthrough," Consumers Union was told by the Bureau of Drugs' associate director for new drug evaluation, Marion J. Finkel, M.D. The official key to the ratings defines A drugs as those that represent "important therapeutic gains" because of increased effectiveness or safety for a disorder not adequately treated by other available drugs.

The designation B means a drug offers a modest but real therapeutic gain over previously licensed products because of greater convenience, elimination of annoying side effects, reduced expense, or less frequent doses. Drugs rated C offer "little or no therapeutic gain," the FDA says.

These classifications thus help to put important information into a succinct, understandable form. A 1-A-rated drug indicates a genuine pharmaceutical advance; a 5-C may mean profit, but certainly not progress. The FDA ratings also can convey additional data:

M—Already marketed outside the U.S.
R—Special conditions of approval apply.
T—Important toxicity problem.
U—Likely to be given to children.

When CU published a sampling of the FDA's ratings of prescription drugs in the October 1978 issue of *Consumer Reports,* it was apparently the first time such information had been made available in print. CU's report drew some criticism from physicians who warned that the ratings could lead, as one put it, to "a great deal of confusion and error in treatment." Understandably some people (including physicians) might assume incorrectly that a rating of A-1 automatically made a drug superior to one with a rating of B-2. Despite some reservations about the format, CU believes that the FDA should make public on a regular basis accurate and complete information about newly approved drugs. The prudent could then protect themselves to some extent from ballyhoo about medical "breakthroughs."

How can you judge a particular piece of news? It usually helps to consider the following six questions. None of the answers may be decisive, but taken all together they can be indicative of the value of the drug.

1. *What is the source of the story?* An announcement from one of the National Institutes of Health or from a major medical center is more likely to be significant than one from the laboratories of a drug firm, however prominent.

2. *Who paid for the study?* Be very critical of the source of funding for the research. Even though some pharmaceutical companies do indeed contribute funds for worthwhile basic research, experimental studies sponsored by drug firms must always be interpreted cautiously or suspected of bias. The same goes for research sponsored by other commercial interests whose motivation for funding studies may be equally self-serving. If government-funded, the research might be valid—or it might not. On some levels of government, political purposes may be served by the premature release of research findings. And the validity of research may be imperiled by changes in policy, which can lead to the elimination or reduction of funds for promising projects. Nevertheless, with government funding, there is more likelihood of disinterest and impartiality. Competition for research grants can be intense, and awards usually go to dependable investigators with promising projects.

Somewhat more reliable as sources of disinterested research are major private foundations (such as Rockefeller or Whitney) that award grants and scholarships to scientists. National health organizations (such as American Heart Association) also sponsor worthwhile research related to their areas of interest. These groups provide many highly qualified investigators with support for quality research in fields allied to the basic interests of the sponsoring organization.

3. *What stage of research is being reported—test tube, animal, or human?* Drug research usually takes place on several different levels of experimentation. A drug's chemical reactions and structural modifications at the molecular level are the particular concerns of basic science. In the next stage, the pharmacological action of the drug on organisms is studied either at the cellular level (which includes viruses and bacteria) or in multicellular organisms (such as rodents and other mammals). Animal experimentation can be scaled to varying degrees of complexity, ranging from use of lower animals, such as rats, to more sophisticated studies with primates. Naturally, the more highly developed the experimental model, the more clinically applicable to humans should be the study results. With drugs that have selective pharmacological action, the organ affected, whether the liver, heart, or kidney, can be removed from the animal and studied as isolated tissue. Only after a drug has been thoroughly studied—not only for physiological effects but also for toxicity—should human experimentation be considered. The final step, clinical testing, involves administering the test drug to humans, according to the provisions of well-designed guidelines provided by the FDA.

Each stage of drug research has its own significance, but the results do not necessarily carry over from one stage to the next. For example, the effects of the drug being studied on isolated rat liver in the test tube may be observed and measured. When the same drug is given to a live rat, however, the effects may not be similar to those noted in vitro. The rat liver in its normal anatomic setting is affected by multiple factors that may reinforce, distort, or otherwise alter the action of the drug under study. Clinical testing is more complicated still. Human beings are more complex than laboratory animals, as well as chemically different in some respects. Furthermore, people have highly developed nervous systems, hence emotions and feelings, which affect them in elaborate and as yet poorly understood ways.

4. *How valid were the clinical testing procedures?* A large proportion of what passes for clinical research is merely old-fashioned trial and error, the results of which are highly vulnerable to false deductions. The reasoning is simple: A drug is given to a sick person; the patient becomes well; therefore the drug is responsible for the cure. The observation that the sick person became well may be accurate, but the deduction that the drug was responsible for the improvement may be false. Illness very often is self-limited—healing or improvement often occurs spontaneously, whether or not medication is prescribed or used.

Even with sound testing procedures, researchers face additional obstacles in clinical trials of drugs. The so-called placebo effect is a well-known phenomenon. As many as 40 percent of participants in some studies report relief of their symptoms when dummy medication has been administered.

Furthermore, results can be distorted by both patient enthusiasm and investigator bias. Just about every sick person wants to get well, and even the most detached investigator wants to come up with a successful result. Both are influenced, perhaps unconsciously, to give the benefit of the doubt to the success of the treatment under study.

Careful investigators attempt to neutralize such factors by resorting to a controlled study—the sound and long-established way to prove or disprove the value of a new medication or treatment. One group of patients receives the drug being tested, and a similar group receives a placebo that looks exactly like the test drug. This method may also utilize a double-blind procedure, in which the drug and the placebo are independently coded so that neither the patients nor the people who administer them and record the results know who receives the drug and who does not. The code is not broken until the study is finished. In addition, the random selection of patients for such tests is important. The experimental and control groups may also be matched in terms of age, gender, and other important variables. Crossover studies, in which drug and placebo are switched without knowledge of patient or observer, also add considerably to test validity.

5. *How extensive was the test?* Of significance here are the number of test subjects, the length of follow-up study of the patients to see how permanent any positive results might be, how serious any long-term side effects might be, and the duration of continued dosage if the drug is for long-term use. The greater each of these has been, the more likely it is that the results will stand up with the passage of time. In this respect it is important to remember that a single study is just that. Ask yourself whether the results of the study have been corroborated by other disinterested investigators.

6. *What does the story report about results and about side effects?* How complete was the cure or relief? Were there risks or side effects and, if so, how serious were they? How do the benefits of the new drug or treatment compare with those of standard measures? Were benefits temporary or long-lasting?

Clear answers to the questions discussed above will help you to evaluate news about drugs, devices, or medical procedures, and to decide whether the label of "miracle" is really warranted.

28

The medicine
cabinet

A few simple, safe, and effective medical supplies, most of them inexpensive, ought to be in any home medicine cabinet. In the following pages Consumers Union's medical consultants recommend everything really needed to meet the common medical problems of most families and to cope with the emergencies most frequently encountered in the home. These supplies need be supplemented only if there are special problems, or if additions are recommended by the family physician.

Drugs to keep on hand

Many bathroom medicine cabinets are a jumble of ancient vials and bottles, some with only a few mysterious tablets. Periodically, check your medicine cabinet and throw out unidentified or outdated prescription medicines and tablets that have disintegrated. At the same time, make sure you have the eight basic over-the-counter (OTC) drugs that CU's medical consultants recommend for the home medicine cabinet: An analgesic/antipyretic, an antacid, an antidiarrheal remedy, an antipruritic, an antiseptic, a decongestant, an emetic, and a laxative. *Remember that any drug is potentially dangerous. All medicines should be stored out of the reach of children.*

Analgesic/antipyretic (see Chapter 1). Buy the least costly aspirin tablets you can find. If you or anyone in your family is allergic to aspirin, acetaminophen may be substituted (see page 27). In homes where aspirin is used mainly for an occasional headache, menstrual cramps, or the aches and pains caused by a cold, a 100-tablet bottle is the size to buy; for more frequent use, buy a larger size. From time to time, check to be sure the tablets have not begun to crumble excessively—which may happen in high-humidity areas. Check also for a strong odor of vinegar. In either case, replacement may be necessary.

For children the usual 5-grain aspirin tablet can be broken easily or cut into halves or quarters to obtain the proper dosage, crushed, and then mixed with applesauce, honey, or jelly.

Parents should think twice before buying children's flavored aspirin. Small children who identify such tablets with candy may be tempted to help themselves. Aspirin in large doses can be fatal. Figures for 1976 show that for children under five about 24 percent of all reported poisoning fatalities were due to swallowing aspirin or other salicylates. Statistics for *ingestion* of aspirin by children less than five years old show that the number of such ingestions has been dropping. In 1973 there were 6,949 cases reported; 5,117 cases were reported in 1974; and the latest figure from the Food and Drug Administration's (FDA) Division of Poison Control was 4,820 in 1976.

So-called tamper-proof caps, required under the poison prevention packaging law of 1972, are helpful but certainly are not perfect prevention. The directives for administering the act say as much: "Special packaging does not mean packaging that all children under five years of age are unable to open or to obtain a harmful amount within a reasonable time." A child who is above-average in dexterity, ingenuity, and persistence, might well open a "tamper-proof" aspirin bottle. Tamper proof or not, precautions must be taken to help prevent ingestion by curious children. A false sense of security could be fatal.

Antacid (see Chapter 7). Sodium bicarbonate is useful for the occasional treatment of heartburn or other symptoms of indigestion—except for those people on a low-sodium diet. If you prefer to use an OTC remedy, read its label carefully; check the list of ingredients to see whether extraneous medication (headache remedies, laxatives, sedatives, etc.) has been added. The closer the product is to a simple antacid, which does nothing more than combat gastric hyperacidity, the better.

Antidiarrheal remedy (see Chapter 8). For diarrhea that may occur from a mild intestinal infection or from a tainted dinner, some people find a kaolin/pectin suspension helpful—even though its efficacy has not yet been proved to the satisfaction of an FDA advisory panel. For those who do not find a kaolin/pectin suspension adequate, or for a more protracted case of diarrhea, a physician should be consulted.

Antipruritic (see Chapter 15). Ordinary calamine lotion can be used for the relief of mild skin eruptions such as mosquito bites, prickly heat, or poison ivy. A compress of cool tap water may also be helpful. (Some prefer to soak in very hot water.)

Antiseptic (see Chapter 14). Isopropyl (70 percent) alcohol —usually purchased as rubbing alcohol—is the only antiseptic normally needed in the home. In most cases, minor wounds can be treated adequately by allowing the wound to bleed a little and then washing gently with soap and water. For more protection, swab the skin around the wound with alcohol, but try not to get alcohol in the wound. Cover with a sterile dressing, if necessary.

Decongestant (see Chapter 2). Phenylephrine hydrochloride solution USP one-half percent may be used as a nasal spray or as nose drops, two or three times a day at most, to reduce the stuffiness of a common cold. This drug deteriorates in storage, so buy only one-half ounce at a time. (Use one-fourth percent solution for infants and children.) An alternative for some might be an oral decongestant (see page 49).

Emetic (see Chapter 17). Most physicians believe that syrup of ipecac (available OTC) should be readily accessible. Poisoning by accidental or intentional ingestion of drugs, household cleansers, and the like may be averted by the oral administration of a vomiting inducer such as ipecac. Emetics should not be used if the swallowed poison is corrosive—for example, lye or strong acid.

Laxative (see Chapter 8). If dietary measures do not bring relief from constipation, it is best to have on hand for occasional use a mild laxative such as methylcellulose, psyllium, or a stool softener such as dioctyl sodium sulfosuccinate.

Home first-aid and sick-room equipment

- *Adhesive bandages,* with plastic-coated gauze that does not stick to a wound. Avoid the tinted medicated type, which may cause an allergic skin reaction.
- *Roll bandage,* 2 inches wide.
- *Sterile gauze pads,* 4 inches square, separately wrapped.
- *Adhesive tape,* one small roll 1 or 2 inches wide.
- *Scissors,* sharp enough to cut gauze or cloth.
- *Tweezers,* with fine points for removing splinters.
- *Elastic bandages,* about 3 inches wide, for wrapping sprained joints. (Be careful not to apply them too tightly.)
- *Ice bag,* to minimize bleeding and also to relieve acute pain resulting from injury to joints and muscles. Cold (*not* heat) should be applied immediately following the injury and then intermittently up to twenty-four hours thereafter, using a towel between the skin and the ice bag. After twenty-four hours, mild heat may be beneficial in reducing swelling. Injured joints should be kept relatively immobile to allow torn tendons and muscles to heal.

- *Hot-water bottle or electric heating pad,* for mild muscular aches. Extreme care should be taken to avoid burning the skin. Never use a heating pad in conjunction with liniment or balm; severe blistering may result.
- *Two clinical thermometers,* one rectal, one oral. Make sure the numerical divisions on the thermometers are easy to read.
- *Enema equipment,* such as prepacked disposable enemas *(Fleet)* can be a convenience although relatively expensive.
- *Electric vaporizer,* for relief of acute respiratory symptoms (see page 55). A child with croup can often find quick relief in a bathroom steamed up by running hot water full force.
- *First-aid manual,* the most comprehensive and authoritative of such publications for the general public is the American National Red Cross's *Standard First Aid and Personal Safety.* A copy may be obtained from local chapters for $1.95. This version of the old *First Aid Textbook* also includes information useful for vacation campers and others who spend much time out in the country or in the woods. And for the first time it includes instructions for foreign body obstruction of the airway (the Heimlich maneuver), first aid for poisoning, and information on how to treat snakebite.
- *Telephone number list,* including both day and night numbers of the family doctor, the nearest poison control center, the pharmacist, the local police or fire department (which often provides emergency services, such as an ambulance or oxygen), and, if available, the volunteer ambulance corps.

Some items *not* recommended

CU's medical consultants believe the following products should be omitted as serving no useful purpose, even though they may be recommended by some authorities or are traditionally included in the medicine cabinet.

- *Antiseptics* (such as *Mercurochrome,* tincture of *Merthiolate,* and similar mercury antiseptics; also tincture of iodine). Ordinary rubbing alcohol is the sensible choice of antiseptic (see Chapter 14).

- *Aromatic spirits of ammonia.* These are frequently recommended for the treatment of fainting. The only necessary thing to do if someone faints is to place the victim in a horizontal position and await recovery. This usually occurs in a minute or two—any period of unconsciousness lasting longer than a few minutes warrants medical attention. Do not force any liquids down the throat of an unconscious or semiconscious person; such heroics may result in a near-drowned victim.

- *Boric acid solutions and powders.* In 1973 Canada prohibited the sale of products containing boric acid or sodium borate to be used as teething preparations or topical applications for infants and children less than three years of age. Canada also requires a warning label on all drugs containing these compounds. CU's medical consultants believe that boric acid solutions and powders offer no medical benefits, and in view of possible toxicity should not be in home medicine cabinets.

- *Cough syrups and elixirs.* Any cough that cannot be relieved within a week by steam inhalation, hot drinks, or sucking hard candies should be checked by a doctor (see Chapter 2).

- *Over-the-counter burn ointments.* They contain anesthetics such as benzocaine, and may cause allergic skin reactions in some people. Instead, the immediate use of ice water or cold running water for the emergency treatment of minor burns should help to minimize pain and retard bleeding (see Chapter 14).

Glossary

This list of medical terms is selected primarily from the pages of *The Medicine Show.* Words and phrases defined here include those occurring in more than one chapter, those indispensable to understanding the material in a chapter, and those that may help clarify some of the definitions themselves. This last criterion is reflected in the frequent use of **bold face** as a guide to other terms in the glossary.

Not listed in the glossary are the names of drugs (over-the-counter and prescription), the names of most diseases, and words adequately defined in the book. Although the definitions can ease reading of *The Medicine Show,* they should also be of help in understanding other references to medical matters.

ABSORPTION. A process by which **drugs** and foods pass through a barrier, such as the intestinal wall or the skin, into the bloodstream.

ACID. A broad category of chemical substances, marked among other things by sour taste and a propensity to react with **alkaline** substances (bases) to form salts. Most bodily functions depend upon the maintenance of a balance between acids and bases in cells, blood, and other body fluids.

(See also **acidification, buffered, neutralizing capacity.**)

ACIDIFICATION (urinary). In a healthy body, **acids** and bases are kept in balance by the excretion of acid in the urine. Certain **drugs** such as ascorbic acid (vitamin C) may increase the concentration of acid in the urine. The ability of the kidneys to excrete acid is impaired by certain diseases.

ACTINIC KERATOSIS. A horny growth on the skin resulting from longstanding exposure to the sun's actinic (ultraviolet) rays.

ACUTE. Describing an illness that comes on suddenly with strong sharp **symptoms** (such illnesses are usually of short duration), or any disease that needs urgent medical attention. (See also **chronic.**)

ADDICTING, ADDICTION. Describing the property of certain **drugs,** such as alcohol, **barbiturates,** and **narcotics,** that leads to compulsive use by some people. Addiction generally manifests itself in three ways: **Tolerance** to the drug develops so that the user no longer obtains the effect achieved with earlier dosage; physical withdrawal **symptoms,** sometimes even life-threatening, occur for a time if use of the addicting drug is curtailed; and recurrent craving for the drug is experienced even long after recovery from withdrawal symptoms.

ADMINISTRATION. The method of introducing a **drug** into a patient's body. It includes dosage (how much), schedule (how often), and route (by mouth, by injection, etc.). (See also **regimen, systemic, topical.**)

ADRENAL GLANDS. A pair of **endocrine** glands, one perched atop each kidney. Among the major products of the adrenal glands' outer or **cortical** layer are the **corticosteroids,** notably **cortisone** and hydrocortisone. The inner core or medulla produces **adrenaline.**

ADRENALINE. A **hormone** secreted by the inner core or

medulla of the **adrenal glands**. It acts on diverse organs and systems of the body to prepare one for "fight or flight," or other stressful situations. It is also available as the **drug** epinephrine (Adrenalin).

ADSORB. See **bind**.

ALKALI, ALKALINE. The chemical opposite of **acid**. Synonym: base. When an alkaline substance reacts with an **acid**, the two **neutralize** each other and form a salt. Lye is a common alkaline substance. (See also **acidification, buffered, neutralizing capacity**.)

ALLERGEN. A substance (usually a protein) that causes an **allergy**.

ALLERGY. A person's abnormal reaction to a substance called an **allergen**. It results from the body's immune mechanism being overwhelmed. **Symptoms** may include runny nose, red and itchy eyes, skin rash, wheezing, or sneezing. These symptoms are usually caused by the release of histamine. (See also **antihistamine, desensitization**.)

AMINO ACIDS. Basic chemical units into which food proteins are broken down during digestion, and from which body proteins are built up in various cells and organs, such as the liver.

ANALGESIC. A **drug**, such as aspirin or codeine, that decreases pain.

ANALOGUE. A chemical **compound** similar in structure to another chemical compound and having the same effect on body processes.

ANAPHYLACTIC, ANAPHYLAXIS. An **acute** allergic response—manifested by cardiovascular collapse—to an **allergen** to which a person has been previously sensitized. Anaphylactic shock can be fatal.

ANATOMIC. Having to do with the shape, structure, and relative position of the body's various parts, as distinct from their function (physiology) or malfunction (pathology).

ANEMIA. A reduction in the number of red blood cells whose function it is to distribute oxygen to all parts of the body. Anemic blood looks "washed out"—how the patient feels.

ANESTHETIC. A **drug** used to deaden pain or to cause loss of consciousness. A local anesthetic dulls sensation at a specific spot or over a small portion of the body; a general anesthetic banishes pain by bringing on a deep artificial sleep; a **topical** anesthetic works only on the area of skin to which it is applied.

ANOREXIA. A **pathological** loss of appetite; aversion to food.

ANTACID. Short for antiacid—an **alkaline compound** that **neutralizes acid,** especially in the stomach.

ANTIBIOTIC. A substance that can kill harmful **microorganisms** in the body, or else keep them from multiplying until the body's own defenses can destroy them. Broad-spectrum antibiotics attack a wide range of germs; narrow-spectrum ones zero in on specific types. Unlike **antiseptics,** antibiotics can be made by living organisms—**fungi**—from which they are extracted and refined for **pharmacological** use. They can also be synthesized in the laboratory.

ANTIBODY. A protein substance made by certain **white blood cells** in the body in response to injection, **ingestion,** or inhalation of an **antigen.** The production of an antibody can be beneficial, as in the case of immunization. (See also **immunological response, vaccine.**)

ANTICOAGULANT. A **drug** used to retard the clotting of blood. Typical anticoagulants are heparin (Meparin, Panheprin) and warfarin (Athrombin-K, Coumadin, Panwarfin).

ANTIGEN. A substance that causes the body's immune system to make a specific **antibody** that will react with (or **neutralize**) that antigen. (See also **immunological response, vaccine.**)

ANTIHISTAMINE. A **drug** used to treat an **allergy** by counteracting the effects of histamine, a chemical manufactured by certain cells in the body.

ANTIHYPERTENSIVE. A drug taken by a person with **hypertension** to lower blood pressure and keep it lowered.

ANTIPRURITIC. A medication used to relieve itching. There are **topical** antipruritics, such as calamine lotion; others are taken by mouth.

ANTIPYRETIC. A **drug,** such as aspirin or acetaminophen, that lowers fever.

ANTISEPTIC. A chemical substance that prevents **infection** by destroying **microorganisms** on the skin, or curtails their multiplication. (See also **antibiotic, germicidal.**)

ASSAY. To analyze and quantify a substance.

ASTRINGENT. A substance that makes blood vessels or other tissues "pucker up" or contract. Alum, the material in styptic pencils, is a typical astringent used to stop small cuts from bleeding.

ASYMPTOMATIC. Without **symptoms;** signifying that an **infection** or disease is in a latent stage, is in **remission,** or simply is cured.

ATONIC. Flaccid, lacking **tone.** When a nerve is injured, the muscle supplied by that nerve becomes atonic. When intestinal muscles are atonic, **peristalsis** is inadequate and constipation results.

ATROPHY. A decrease in size and function of a part of the body from lack of use or from disruption of nerve supply, blood flow, or **hormone** delivery to that part of the body.

BACTERIA. General name for a vast variety of **microorganisms,** including beneficial as well as harmful types. "Good" bacteria make yogurt, aid digestion, and help to nourish growing plants. "Bad" or disease-producing bacteria cause all manner of infectious diseases.

BACTERIAL RESISTANCE. When a person acquires **immunity** against a strain of **bacteria,** that's good. But when the bacteria develop immunity of their own against an **antibiotic,** that's resistance—and that's bad.

BARBITURATE. A type of **drug** used in small doses as a **sedative,** and in larger doses as a **hypnotic.** Barbiturates can be **addicting.**

BELLADONNA ALKALOIDS. A mixture of plant derivatives including atropine, scopolamine, and related chemicals. As a group, the belladonna alkaloids work against the **parasympathetic nervous system.** One of their actions is to dry **secretions** of the **mucous membranes** in the mouth, nose, and stomach.

BIND (ADSORB). To enter into a chemical bond, as when one substance unites or combines firmly with another.

BIOCHEMICAL. Having to do with the chemical composition of the body as well as its **metabolism,** rather than its anatomy or physiology.

BIOPSY. Surgical removal of a small slice or sliver of tissue for examination, usually under a microscope, to see if its cells are cancerous or otherwise abnormal.

BLIND TRIAL. A **controlled trial** of a **drug** in which the patients do not know whether they are being given the real thing or a **placebo**—but their doctors know. (See also **double-blind trial.**)

BONE MARROW FAILURE. Marrow, the soft pith or filling inside bones, manufactures the blood's red cells (which deliver oxygen throughout the body), **white cells** (which fight **infection**), and platelets (which help **clotting**). Certain **drugs,** as well as radiation, damage marrow so it cannot produce these cells; the phenomenon that results is bone marrow failure. Bone marrow failure may be partial, affecting only one type of blood cell rather than all three.

BRONCHI. Plural of bronchus; subdivisions of the trachea (windpipe), which further subdivide into bronchioles (narrower and narrower air tubes) descending deep into the lungs. Bronchitis is the name for **inflammation** of the bronchi.

BUFFERED. Describing therapeutic preparations to which **antacids** have been added. In the case of aspirin, buffering ostensibly protects the stomach against the corrosive effect of the aspirin.

CAPILLARY. The very finest subdivision of the body's network of blood vessels, the capillary is a microscopic blood vessel, much finer than a hair, with ultra-thin walls, through which the blood gives up its oxygen to the body's tissues.

CARCINOGENIC. Cancer-causing. (See also **mutagenic**.)

CARRIER. In **drugs** and cosmetics, the (relatively) **inert** substance in which the active ingredient is dissolved, mixed, or suspended for ease of **administration**.

CENTRAL NERVOUS SYSTEM. The brain and spinal cord together serve as a command module that governs branching networks of peripheral nerves and the **sympathetic nervous system**. The central nervous system also controls thinking, dreaming, and consciousness.

CHEMICAL CAUTERIZATION. A burning away of unwanted living tissue (warts, for example) by means of caustic **compounds,** such as strong **acids** or **alkalies.**

CHEMOTHERAPY. Treatment of disease (**therapy**) by medicating with chemical **compounds**. Synonym: **drug** therapy.

CHROMOSOMES. The thousands of genes that carry hereditary messages from parents to offspring are strung on forty-six microscopic "necklaces" called chromosomes. The chromosomes are tightly coiled inside most body cells, including sperm and ova. These strings of **genetic** beads can

be broken and partly lost or wrongly restrung by certain
chemicals, infectious agents, radiation, and other factors—
thus causing birth defects.

CHRONIC. Describing a disease of long duration or one that
is recurrent. (See also **acute.**)

CLINICAL. Having to do with the medical care of ill people,
and treatment of their signs and **symptoms,** as distinct from
experimentation with laboratory animals. Thus a clinical
trial involves trying new **therapy** on human subjects.

CLINICIAN. A practicing physician. Besides treating sick
people, the clinician may (or may not) teach medicine and
take part in medical research.

CLOTTING MECHANISM. The body's self-sealing system.
When blood is shed, a complex series of **biochemical** reactions starts. The process ends with the manufacture of a
tough substance called fibrin, which closes the wound and
stops the bleeding. Certain **anticoagulants,** such as heparin
(Meparin, Panheprin) and warfarin (Athrombin-K, Coumadin, Panwarfin), can disrupt this clotting or **coagulation**
mechanism. Aspirin is also an anticlotting agent by dint of
its effects on platelets. The clotting mechanism is lacking in
people afflicted with clotting factor deficiencies such as
hemophilia.

COAGULATION. What happens to the white of an egg
when it's boiled. A complex **biochemical** process by which
the blood forms solid clumps or clots to staunch a bleeding
wound and thus start the healing process. (See also **thrombosed.**)

COMPOUND. In medical parlance, a preparation formed by
combining several ingredients according to a formula. In
chemical terms, a uniform substance formed by the stable
combination of two or more chemical elements, as distinct
from a mere mixture. (See also **molecular structure.**)

CONGENITAL. Present at birth and usually arising during the **fetus's** development in the uterus. Congenital defects or malformations are either **genetic**—inherited from one or both parents—or produced during pregnancy (as by a **drug** the woman may have used) or resulting from a **virus** or other **infection** the pregnant woman may have acquired and passed on to the **embryo** or fetus.

CONGESTION. The disruption of function in certain parts of the body by swelling of the lining tissues and by partial obliteration of the normal channels of blood flow or air flow. For instance, in **congestive heart failure,** congestion of the lungs occurs, making breathing arduous. Nasal congestion means swelling of the **mucous membranes** of the nose, making breathing through the nose difficult.

CONGESTIVE HEART FAILURE. A disorder characterized by swelling of the ankles and by shortness of breath. Congestive heart failure may follow a heart attack when the heart muscle has been severely damaged and thus can no longer function efficiently as a pump. Heart failure may also result from other forms of heart disease or from lung disease. (See also **coronary heart disease.**)

CONNECTIVE TISSUE. The "cement" of the body in which most cells are embedded. Connective tissue is made up for the most part of a material called collagen. Certain diseases, such as rheumatoid arthritis (see **rheumatology**), rheumatic fever, and lupus erythematosus, are disorders that primarily affect collagen.

CONTRAINDICATION. A reason not to use a given medication in a given situation; for example, many ordinarily beneficial **drugs** are contraindicated during pregnancy.

CONTROLLED SUBSTANCES. Within the context of this book, certain **prescription drugs,** such as **analgesics,** that are **addicting** and for which physicians and druggists must record and report every prescription in order to prevent illicit traffic and abuse.

CONTROLLED TRIAL or STUDY. When a **drug** or other form of **therapy** is tried out **clinically,** to determine its efficacy, **toxicity, side effects,** indications, and **contraindications,** variable factors that could distort these results must be minimized. This is done by comparing the response of a trial group (patients who receive the new treatment) with that of a group of control subjects (patients who do not). The trial group and the control group are carefully matched for similarity in age, gender, and other relevant factors. (See also **blind trial, double-blind trial.**)

CORONARY HEART DISEASE. The name for the disorder that results from reduction in blood flow to the heart muscle due to narrowing of the coronary arteries by accumulation of fatty substances in the walls of the arteries. Activities that increase the heart rate can then cause transient chest pains (known as angina pectoris). If a narrowed coronary artery becomes completely blocked by a blood clot (coronary thrombosis), the portion of the heart muscle supplied by that artery usually ceases to function. This is known as a heart attack—technically, myocardial infarction. (See also **congestive heart failure.**)

CORROSIVE. Capable of destroying tissue, as a strong **acid** or **alkali.**

CORTICAL. Referring to the outer layer of certain organs. For instance, the cortical layer of the **adrenal glands** (adrenal cortex) secretes **corticosteroids.**

CORTICOSTEROID. A family of potent, versatile **hormones** originating mainly in the **adrenal glands,** used therapeutically to treat **inflammatory** and allergic diseases. A corticosteroid can be produced naturally in the adrenal glands or synthesized in the laboratory.

CORTISONE. A **corticosteroid** that can be made in the body or synthesized in the laboratory. Introduced in 1952, this chemical is useful in treating many diseases but may have serious long-term **side effects**.

CULTURE. A method of growing cells or **microorganisms** in the laboratory in order to identify them and to determine their resistance to **antibiotics**. The special food on which they are grown is the culture **medium**. (See also **in vitro, in vivo.**)

CYCLIC. Repeating on a regular periodic on-again, off-again schedule.

DECONGESTANT. A substance—usually a **vasoconstrictor** —that relieves nasal **congestion**.

DEGENERATIVE. Referring to changes in bodily function that reflect deterioration of certain cells or tissues, and the substances they secrete. For example, osteoarthritis is a degenerative joint disease.

DEHYDRATION. Loss of water from the body or any of its tissues, beyond normal sweating and urination. If mild, it triggers thirst to restore the fluid balance; if severe and sudden (for example, as a result of massive diarrhea), dehydration can cause shock and death, especially in young children.

DEMULCENT. A substance that soothes, softens, or protects a **mucous membrane** surface. An **emollient** does the same for skin.

DEPENDENCE. Can be physical or psychological. Physical dependence is synonymous with **addiction**. Psychological dependence may be equated with the **placebo** effect.

DEPRESSANT. A **drug**, such as a **barbiturate** or alcohol, that acts on the **central nervous system** to diminish mental acuity and muscular activity.

DERMATITIS. An **inflammation** of the skin due to any of many causes, known and unknown. Thus, contact dermatitis is a rash occurring as a reaction to some irritating chemical, textile, or other material touching or rubbing the skin. (See also **eczema**.)

DESENSITIZATION. A process by which **allergy** is reduced by periodic injection of gradually increasing amounts of the offending **allergen**. A more accurate term for this process is hyposensitization because complete desensitization is rarely achieved.

DETOXIFY. To remove or neutralize the harmful activity of a **toxic** substance in the body.

DIABETES MELLITUS. An all-too-familiar disorder of **metabolism,** in which the body cannot assimilate sugar for lack —or relative lack—of the pancreatic **hormone** insulin. Popularly shortened to diabetes.

DIATHERMY. Deep heat **therapy,** generated by microwaves, aimed at muscles and joints. A microwave oven uses a similar principle.

DIGITALLY. Refers to an examination technique in which the physician uses a finger (as in a rectal examination).

DIURETIC. A **drug** that acts to eliminate fluid from the body by increasing the amount of urine released.

DOUBLE-BLIND TRIAL. A **controlled trial** of a **drug** in a **clinical** situation in which neither the recipients nor the experimenters (hence: double) know which patients are receiving the active substance, and which are being given a **placebo.** This dual ignorance minimizes subjective reactions to the drug being tested. (See also **blind trial**.)

DRUG. Medical meaning: Any chemical agent or medicinal substance (**compound,** preparation, remedy, etc.) used to promote health or to treat disease by causing a desired change within the body or on its surface. Popular meaning: Certain chemical compounds and plant substances that alter mood or mental or emotional state; some of these drugs are **addicting.**

DUODENAL ULCER. When the highly **acid** gastric juices of the stomach eat away at the wall of the duodenum (the first part of the small intestine below the stomach), the resulting raw sore is a duodenal ulcer. A duodenal ulcer can be painful and can bleed. If the ulcer heals with excessive scar tissue, an intestinal obstruction may result. (See also **peptic ulcer.**)

ECZEMA. A type of **dermatitis,** usually caused by an **allergy.**

ELECTROENCEPHALOGRAPHIC. Relating to the electroencephalograph (EEG)—a machine that helps a neurologist diagnose brain **tumors,** epilepsy, and other disorders by detecting abnormalities in the electrical waves emanating from different areas of the brain. Similar to the electrocardiograph (ECG)—a machine that helps a physician detect electrical impulses from the heart.

ELIXIR. A liquid form of the sugar-coated pill. A mixture of water, sweetener, scent, and alcohol, used as a **carrier** to make medicine pleasant tasting.

EMBRYO. The earliest stage of human development in the uterus from the time the ovum has been fertilized until about two months later. (See also **fetus.**)

EMETIC. A substance that provokes vomiting when swallowed.

EMOLLIENT. A substance—such as petrolatum or olive oil —that soothes, softens, or protects the skin surface. A **demulcent** does the same for **mucous membrane.**

ENDOCRINE SYSTEM. An interlocking directorate of glands whose **hormones** control bodily growth, sex characteristics, **metabolism,** and many other functions. The main endocrine glands are the **adrenals,** ovaries, pancreas, parathyroids, **pituitary,** testes, and thyroid.

ENTITY. A specifically defined thing, usually said of a particular **molecular structure** or a characteristic disease.

ENZYMES. Proteins made by the body that act as catalysts for many **biochemical** reactions. Enzymes also break down food and other substances into simpler chemical **compounds** that can then be absorbed, metabolized, or otherwise used by the body. Enzymes are also used commercially; meat tenderizer, for instance, is an enzyme.

EUPHORIA. In medical terms, an exaggerated feeling of well-being or elation.

EXPECTORATING, EXPECTORATION, EXPECTORANT. Coughing up and spitting out of phlegm (see also **exudate**) from the lungs and **bronchi.** An expectorant is a substance that eases coughing and makes the **sputum** less thick.

EXUDATE (PUS). A thick fluid containing dead **white blood cells, microorganisms,** and solid cellular debris that oozes or leaks from the blood into tissues at the site of an **infection.**

FETUS. The product of conception after graduating from its first two months of life as an **embryo** and until it becomes an infant at birth.

FOLIC ACID. A nutrient used by the **bone marrow** in the production of red blood cells.

FREE FATTY ACID. An organic **acid** "freed" from a more complex **compound** (triglyceride) in the **metabolism** of body fat.

FUNCTIONAL DISEASE. A disorder due to the faulty working of one or more structurally healthy organs or parts of the body. As opposed to **organic disease.**

FUNGUS. A parasitic **microorganism,** best known as the itchy villain in athlete's foot. The category also includes some medically more important types that infect internal organs and can even cause death. Some fungi, though, are beneficial—such as the molds that produce **antibiotics,** and the yeast that makes bread rise.

GASTROINTESTINAL. Having to do with the digestive tract including the esophagus, stomach, small intestine, large intestine, and rectum. Abbreviated "GI" (as in GI series, which is an X-ray visualization of the upper part of the gastrointestinal tract taken after the patient swallows a radiopaque substance, such as barium).

GEL. A substance of jelly-like consistency.

GENERIC. Describing the name given to a **drug** by the United States Adopted Names Council (see Chapter 25), as distinct from the registered brand name a pharmaceutical company gives to its version of the same preparation.

GENETIC. Inherited through the parents' genes. Genetic traits (such as color of hair and eyes), as well as genetic diseases and defects, run in families in more or less predictable patterns. A child inherits traits and characteristics, as well as defects or susceptibility to certain diseases. Such genetic effects may not be readily noticeable in the parents; they are passed on by union of the parental ovum and sperm, rather than by what happens during pregnancy.

GENITOURINARY. Genital plus urinary equal genitourinary. The body's reproduction and urinary system, extending from kidneys to ureters, bladder, and **urethra** (that is, the urinary tract), plus the adjacent genital tract. In males, the latter runs from testes to prostate and penis; in females, from ovaries, Fallopian tubes, and uterus to cervix and vagina.

GERMICIDAL. Referring to chemical agents—lethal to germs—which are generally used on inanimate objects (i.e., germicidal solutions for sterilizing surgical instruments). Describes the action of certain **antiseptics.** (See also **microorganisms.**)

GLAUCOMA. A serious eye disease caused by buildup of fluid pressure inside the eyeball. Part of the **degenerative** aging process, simple or **chronic** glaucoma usually comes on gradually; if untreated, it usually destroys the optic nerve, causing blindness. Closed-angle (also known as narrow-angle) or **acute** glaucoma has a sudden severe onset due to narrowing of the eyeball's natural drainage channels. Acute glaucoma is accompanied by severe pain. If untreated, acute glaucoma can lead to irreparable damage.

GLUTEN. A protein in wheat and other grains that is thought to produce a special **allergy** in susceptible people, with unpleasant digestive effects including cramps and diarrhea. A gluten-free diet is helpful in celiac disease and nontropical sprue.

GRAIN. The apothecary's traditional unit of weight—approximately $65/1000$ of a **gram**. It is still used by doctors in prescribing—and by pharmacists in compounding—pills, powders, and potions. (See also **milligram**.)

GRAM. A unit of weight in the metric system, often used to measure **drugs**. Approximately 28 grams equal 1 ounce; $1/1000$ of a gram is a **milligram**. (See also **grain**.)

GRAM-NEGATIVE and -POSITIVE. **Bacteria** are of two varieties: Gram-positive bacteria are visible under the microscope when dyed by a certain technique—Gram's stain; Gram-negative bacteria fail to hold the color. (Named after Hans Gram, a Danish bacteriologist, not after the **gram** unit of weight.)

GRANULOMAS. Microscopic **lesions** composed of whorls of **inflammatory** tissue. Granuolmas are present in such diseases as **sarcoidosis**, tuberculosis, and certain fungal **infections**.

HALLUCINOGEN. A **drug** that may cause some individuals to see or hear things that really aren't real.

HALOGENS. A group of related chemical elements—chlorine, iodine, bromine, and fluorine. They combine readily with hydrogen to form **acids,** and with metals to form salts.

HEMOLYTIC. Referring to the process of hemolysis by which the membrane surrounding a red blood cell breaks. Hemolysis may be caused by a defect in the red cell membrane itself (as in sickle cell **anemia**) or by an **antibody** that clings to and damages the red cell membrane.

HEMORRHAGE. Excessive loss of blood from the body or into its inner cavities through cut or torn veins, arteries, or **capillaries.**

HORMONE. A chemical substance made in an **endocrine** gland and secreted into the bloodstream. The hormone then acts on some distant target within the body.

HOST. (1) An organism (especially a human being) in and on which an invading **microorganism** thrives. (2) An individual who receives a donor transplant organ.

HOUSE STAFF. Medical doctors enrolled in a hospital training program; popularly referred to as interns and residents.

HYPER-. A prefix meaning more than normal.

HYPERTENSION. A disorder that is characterized by increased blood pressure. If undetected or untreated, hypertension may eventually affect the functioning of the brain, eyes, heart, and kidneys.

HYPNOTIC. A **drug** that induces sleep. Some hypnotics, in smaller dosage, are used as **sedatives.**

HYPO-. A prefix meaning less than normal.

IDIOPATHIC. A medical term used to describe a disease of unknown cause or origin.

IMMUNE MECHANISM. See **immunological response.**

IMMUNITY. Resistance to a specific **infection.** (See also **vaccine.**)

IMMUNOLOGICAL RESPONSE. The production of specific proteins called **antibodies** by certain **white blood cells**

in response to stimulation by specific **antigens** (e.g., **bacteria, viruses,** pollens). The antibodies resist in varying degrees invasion of the body by these **microorganisms** and other alien substances. Transfused blood of the wrong type or an organ transplanted from another body can also induce this response.

INCIDENCE. In general, the frequency with which something happens. In particular, the rate at which disease or death occurs in a population; it is usually expressed as so many per hundred thousand individuals. Prevalence, on the other hand, is the total number of cases in an entire population. (See also **mortality.**)

INCUBATE. To facilitate growth or multiplication of cells or germs in a **culture medium (in vitro)** to the point where they can be identified, or **in vivo** to the point where they cause **symptoms.**

INERT. Without physiological action or effect, as a **placebo.**

INFECTION. (1) Invasion of the body, or one of its parts, by a harmful **microorganism.** (2) The disease thus caused by the invasion.

INFLAMMATION. The body's four-alarm response to injury or infection: (1) pain (2) heat (3) reddening and (4) swelling. These local reactions signify that the body is rallying its forces to limit and repair the damage. Inflammation is thus not the same as **infection,** although the latter often triggers inflammation.

INGESTED, INGESTION. Swallowed, taken by mouth into the **gastrointestinal** tract. Ingestion is the most common mode of **administration** for **drugs**—pills, powders, potions, capsules, syrups, **elixirs,** etc. Other methods include injection into bloodstream, muscle or skin, infusion, inhalation, and **absorption.**

INSULT. Any injury, abuse, maltreatment or excessive stress suffered by a cell, tissue, organ—or entire body. (See also **reversible.**)

IN VITRO. Literally, "in glass"—a medical or biological event that takes place, outside the human body, in the laboratory. As opposed to **in vivo.** (See also **culture, incubate.**)

IN VIVO. Literally, "in life"—a medical or biological event that takes place in a living human or animal. As opposed to **in vitro.** (See also **culture, incubate.**)

IODIDE. Derived from iodine, a **halogen.** Iodide-containing salts such as sodium iodide or potassium iodide. Iodide that is **ingested** in food or medication is avidly picked up by the thyroid gland where it is used for the manufacture of thyroid **hormones.** Radioactive iodide is often used to diagnose and treat certain thyroid diseases. (See also **radioactive isotope.**)

IONIZING RADIATION. High-energy radiation, such as that produced by X rays, gamma rays from **radioactive isotopes,** and nuclear fallout, which penetrate deep into bodily tissue. In high enough doses, ionizing radiation, precisely aimed at **tumor** cells, may kill or cripple them. But at the same time, healthy cells in its path may suffer **inflammation,** death, or transformation into malignant cells.

IRREVERSIBLE. A medical term for incurable. A one-way process of deterioration that may be arrested, perhaps, but never cured.

-ITIS. A suffix meaning **inflammation** of, as in appendicitis.

LACTATING. Producing breast milk, as a mother who breast-feeds her baby.

LESION. Any damaged site or local **pathological** condition in skin or internal tissue, caused by disease, degeneration, or injury.

MEDIUM. What **bacteria** feed on—the special mixture of nutrients, chemical, and fluids in which and on which **cul-**

tured cells and **microorganisms** grow in laboratories.

MEMBRANE. See **mucous membrane.**

METABOLISM. The **biochemical** processes by which food and oxygen are used by the body to provide the energy that is necessary for the proper functioning of body organs and tissues.

METABOLITE. A new substance formed in the body by **metabolism** of a given **drug** or chemical. It may act quite differently from the original substance, its **precursor.**

MICROORGANISMS. Living creatures too small to be seen with the naked eye. **Pathological** microorganisms, which cause **infections** in larger forms of life, are known colloquially as germs. They include **viruses, bacteria,** and **fungi.**

MILLIGRAM. $\frac{1}{1000}$ of a gram; a unit of weight in the metric system of measurement, in which **drug** dosages can be measured. (See also **grain, gram.**)

MOLECULAR STRUCTURE. The architecture of a **compound.** By making small changes in the molecular structure of a **drug, analogues** are produced and the **pharmacological** effects of the original substance may be altered.

MORTALITY. The statistical rate at which people die of a given cause, usually expressed as so many deaths per hundred thousand people. (Morbidity, on the other hand, is the rate at which people get sick from a specific cause.)

MUCOUS MEMBRANE. The body's "inside skin"—extremely thin, soft layers of cells that line the surface of certain body tracts such as the **respiratory** tract and the **gastrointestinal** tract.

MUCUS. A colorless substance secreted by the **mucous** cells of the intestines, cervix, and **respiratory** tract.

MUTAGENIC. Able to alter the **genetic** message by which a given cell reproduces its kind. Such a mutation of the cell may result in cancer; the mutagenic substance is then said to be **carcinogenic** as well. Or, if the mutated cells are in the reproductive system, they may cause birth defects.

NARCOTIC. A natural or synthetic **addicting drug** used medically to relieve pain or to produce sleep by depressing the **central nervous system.** Examples are codeine, meperidine (Demerol), and morphine.

NEPHROLOGY. A branch of medical science dealing with the kidney—its structure, functions, and diseases.

NEUTRAL, NEUTRALIZE. Any substance that is neither **acid** nor **alkaline** is said to be neutral. When an acid meets an alkaline substance in a test tube or the stomach, for instance, they neutralize each other to form a salt.

NEUTRALIZING CAPACITY. The ability of an **alkali** to offset acidity. (See also **antacid.**)

NF. Refers to a **drug** compounded according to the *National Formulary,* a semiofficial directory of drug standards and specifications, issued every five years by the American Pharmaceutical Association. (See also **USP.**)

NODULAR THYROID. A thyroid gland that has one or more lumps that can be felt through the skin of the neck. A nodular thyroid requires evaluation by a physician.

NOSTRUM. A "remedy" for which extravagant, scientifically unsupported therapeutic claims are often made; a **patent medicine.**

OCCLUSION. In general, the closing or blocking of a blood vessel or some other passageway or orifice in the body. In dentistry, the manner in which upper and lower teeth meet when the jaws shut; the "bite."

ONCOLOGY. A branch of medical science dealing with **tumors** (particularly cancers)—their origin, nature, growth, effects, and treatment.

ORGANIC DISEASE. A disorder due to **anatomic** changes in a body organ that interferes with an organ's ability to do its job. As opposed to **functional disease** of a structurally intact organ. For example, rectal cancer, an organic disease, may cause constipation. Constipation triggered by a family crisis would be a functional type of bowel disorder.

OVERT. Apparent to the senses; noticeable to a patient or a physician. The opposite of **asymptomatic.**

OVER-THE-COUNTER (OTC) DRUG. A drug that the Food and Drug Administration (FDA) accepts as safe for self-medication. According to the FDA, an OTC drug can be used by consumers for disorders they diagnose themselves and treat by following the directions on the label without advice from a physician. (See also **prescription drug.**)

PARASYMPATHETIC NERVOUS SYSTEM. A network of nerves that controls such involuntary, unconscious, automatic body reactions as dilatation of certain blood vessels, slowdown in heartbeat, narrowing of pupils, salivation, and increased nasal **secretion.** The **sympathetic nervous system** generally has opposite effects.

PATENT MEDICINE. An **over-the-counter** preparation whose formula is usually a trade secret, and for which unproven therapeutic benefits are often claimed; a **nostrum.**

PATHOLOGICAL. Describing an abnormality usually caused by disease.

PEPTIC ULCER. A raw, sore, eroded area on the wall of the stomach or duodenum. When the wall of the stomach or duodenum is eaten all the way through, the **lesion** is called a perforation. If a blood vessel is eroded in the process, bleeding occurs—hence the familiar bleeding ulcer.

PERFORATION (of ulcer). See **peptic ulcer.**

PERINATAL. Referring to the time period from birth to approximately one month afterward.

PERIPHERAL NERVE. A nerve that transmits pain or other sensory perceptions from the skin or limbs to the **central**

nervous system, and sends the brain's messages back out again to these remote—that is, peripheral—parts of the body.

PERISTALSIS. Synchronized, sequential contractions of special muscles in the **gastrointestinal** tract that nudge and squeeze food through the esophagus and stomach to the intestine and rectum.

PHARMACOLOGICAL. Concerning the action—therapeutic or **toxic** or both—of a **drug** on or in the body; its **absorption, metabolism,** and excretion, as well as its effect on cells, tissues, organs, and bodily function.

PHOTOSENSITIVITY REACTION. A heightened sensitivity of the skin to the rays of the sun, caused by certain oral medications or cosmetics.

PHYTATES. Chemical substances, salts of phytic acid, which have the capacity to combine with calcium and iron, thus impairing the body's **absorption** of these nutrients.

PITUITARY. An **endocrine** gland located at the base of the brain: The body's main command module. Its **hormones** direct the activities of the **adrenal glands,** ovaries, testes, and thyroid, and also govern such key processes as growth and **metabolism.**

PLACEBO. A medically **inert** substance formulated to mimic —in color and form—an active substance; used in testing the efficacy of a **drug.** The patients in a **blind trial** (and their doctors, as well, in a **double-blind trial**) do not know who receives the active substance, or who receives the dummy one. In some **clinical** studies as many as 40 percent of the subjects respond favorably to a placebo.

PRECURSOR. That which comes before. Refers to (1) a chemical substance that is converted to another chemical substance (thus, flurazepam is the precursor of its long-lived **metabolite**); or (2) a previously existing disorder that leads to a disease (cystic hyperplasia may be a precursor of endometrial cancer).

PRESCRIPTION DRUG. A **drug** available only by a doctor's prescription; too potent or dangerous or **addicting** to be sold over the counter.

PRESSOR AGENTS. Chemicals (usually **drugs**) that have the effect of raising blood pressure. (See also **vasomotor**.)

PROPELLANT. A gas or liquified gas used to provide the pressure necessary to expel the contents in a self-spraying container.

PROPHYLACTIC, PROPHYLAXIS. Preventive: Tending to guard against or forestall disease by removing its cause, or denying it a chance to develop.

PROSTHETIC, PROSTHESIS. Any artificial or "bionic" device fitted to replace or reinforce a missing or faulty part of the body—for example, a dental crown or a stainless steel hip joint.

PROTOCOL. A plan specifying the rules and regulations for conducting any scientific study. For a **clinical** trial, a protocol lays down such conditions as how many patients will be treated by what means for how long in what manner. (See also **blind trial, double-blind trial, placebo**.)

PSYCHOSIS. One of a group of serious mental or emotional disorders, notably **schizophrenia** and manic-depressive psychosis, which may impair mental functioning sufficiently to interfere with capacity to meet the ordinary demands of life.

PSYCHOSOMATIC. Referring to a group of physical ailments that are known to be caused by emotional factors. These are not imagined illnesses, but conditions in which actual evidence of physical disease can be documented. For example, irritable colon syndrome, bronchial asthma, and **peptic ulcer** are usually considered psychosomatic illnesses.

PSYCHOTHERAPEUTIC DRUG. A chemical **compound**

that is prescribed by a physician in the treatment of mental or emotional disorders.

PSYCHOTHERAPY. The treatment of mental or emotional disorders primarily by interaction between therapist and patient, or therapist and a group of patients, or interaction among patients without a therapist. Its methods include suggestion, persuasion, hypnosis, dream analysis, free-association analysis, and the like.

PULMONARY. Having to do with the lungs.

PUS. See **exudate**.

RADIOACTIVE ISOTOPE. A kind of chemical element, either natural or made in a nuclear reactor, that emits energy in the form of radiation that can be detected by instruments. The isotope of a particular element can mimic its natural counterpart in body **metabolism**. As a result, certain chemical **compounds** "tagged" with the radioactive isotope can be swallowed or injected and followed through the body by a radiation detector making possible many kinds of diagnostic tests. Large doses of radioactive isotopes may be used therapeutically.

REBOUND EFFECT. An intense flare-up of **symptoms** related to the use of medication that occurs when the medication is suddenly withdrawn or its effects wear off. The rebound symptoms are generally more severe than those for which the medication was originally taken. In order to suppress these symptoms the patient may resort to more frequent use of the medication or increased dosage or both. The rebound effect most commonly occurs with the use of nose drops. It also occurs with abrupt discontinuance of **corticosteroids** and occasionally other oral medications.

REFLEX. An automatic, involuntary action of a muscle in response to nerve stimulation. An unconditioned reflex is one built into the nervous system of every normal human being (e.g., the knee-jerk reaction). A conditioned reflex is one that has been learned by experience (e.g., a dog drooling at the sound of a dinner bell).

REGIMEN. Just what the doctor orders; any therapeutic program or schedule for eating, sleeping, exercising, taking medicine, and so forth.

REGURGITATE. To vomit; throw up.

REMISSION. Temporary absence of signs and **symptoms** of a disease, usually an incurable one.

RESISTANT. Immune to or unaffected by. (See also **bacterial resistance.**)

RESPIRATORY. Refers to the body's breathing apparatus: The air passages extending from mouth and nostrils down through the throat and trachea to the **bronchi** and lungs.

RETROSPECTIVE. By hindsight: Conclusions derived from past experience to estimate future results. Prospective means setting up observations or experiments ahead of time to study future events as they happen. Thus, a retrospective **clinical** trial may involve analyses of many case histories in a hospital's files while a prospective study records how patients respond to a **protocol** set up in advance.

REVERSIBLE. Curable; capable of recovering from all signs of illness, injury, or disability. Its opposite, "irreversible" means permanent damage.

RHEUMATIC. Having to do with rheumatism—sore, stiff, inflamed joints and muscles due to various causes, known and unknown.

RHEUMATOLOGY. A branch of medical science dealing with **rheumatic** diseases (such as rheumatoid arthritis and gout) or diseases of **connective tissue.**

SALICYLATES. A class of **compounds** (of which aspirin is the best known) used to relieve pain, reduce **inflammation,** and lower body temperature.

SARCOIDOSIS. A generalized disorder in which **granulomas** develop in various organs of the body, primarily the lungs, but also the liver, lymph nodes, and spleen. The cause of sarcoidosis is unknown. Severe cases are treated with a **corticosteroid.**

SCHIZOPHRENIA. One of a group of **psychoses,** in which the affected person undergoes personality changes marked by withdrawal and bizarre behavior. Hallucinations, delusions, and paranoia are not uncommon.

SCREENING TEST. A mass examination of a large group designed to detect a particular disease early enough to treat it with maximum effect.

SEBUM. A thick greasy **exudate;** a normal **secretion** of the sebaceous glands of skin and scalp.

SECONDARY INFECTION. An **infection** that flares up in a tissue or organ made vulnerable by a prior infection. For example, **bacteria** may secondarily infect a fever blister originally caused by a **virus.**

SECRETION. The product of a gland or glands in the body. An external secretion (usually a complex mixture of organic chemicals) is produced by a nonendocrine gland and is ultimately extruded onto the body's surface; e.g., **sebum** is the secretion of a sebaceous gland; **mucus** is the secretion of **respiratory** or **gastrointestinal** glands; tears are the secretion of the lacrymal glands. An internal secretion, usually a **hormone,** is delivered directly into the bloodstream from its site of manufacture in one of the glands of the **endocrine system.**

SEDATIVE. A **drug** that exerts a calming or quieting effect on mental processes or nervous irritability. (See also **hypnotic, tranquilizer.**)

SENSITIZATION. Stimulation of the body's **immunological response** "memory" by a foreign substance, so that the next time the alien material makes contact—which may be even years later—**symptoms** of the **allergy** may appear.

SERUM FACTORS. In the serum (the liquid part of the blood) there are various types of **antibodies** that help the **white blood cells** to overwhelm infecting **microorganisms.** Serum factors may also be associated with certain diseases such as rheumatoid arthritis (see **rheumatology**) or thyroiditis.

SHOTGUN REMEDY. A medication combining two or more different therapeutic **drugs** in a single preparation, presumably based on the theory that if enough ingredients are used, one might work.

SIDE EFFECT. The cloud inside the silver lining. Every **drug,** along with its desired **pharmacological** action, causes other gratuitous consequences, ranging from incidental to downright **toxic.** Because these dividends—usually unwelcome—may be dose-related, proper **chemotherapy** must specify the exact quantity of **drugs** that offers the best trade-off between benefit and burden to the body.

SIGN. See **symptom.**

SITZ BATH. Fundamental bliss: A warm bath, with or without added salts, in which a patient sits with hips and buttocks under water. Sitz means "seat" in German.

SMEAR. A sample of blood, **mucus,** pus, or other material from the body spread on a glass slide for staining and examination under a microscope.

SODIUM. One of the two chemical elements in table salt (the other is chlorine). In the body, sodium is one of the most important constitutents of blood and of other body fluids. People with **congestive heart failure** or **hypertension** may be advised to reduce sodium in their diet.

SPASM. Involuntary contraction (clenching, tensing, or tightening up) of muscles.

SPECTRUM. Assortment, array. Originally described the range of wavelengths—the rainbow in the sky spanning the spectrum of visible colors. Now refers to any range or span or set of effects, such as a broad-spectrum **antibiotic,** which is effective against both **Gram-positive** and **Gram-negative bacteria** or a variety of disease **symptoms.**

SPHINCTER. A round muscle encircling an opening in the body; when it contracts, it is capable of closing the orifice.

SPUTUM. Mucus, sometimes mixed with pus, coughed up from the lungs and **bronchi.** Synonym: phlegm.

STEROIDS. A family of organic **compounds,** or their **analogues,** of which the **corticosteroid hormones** secreted by the **adrenal glands** are a subdivision. Steroids perform a vital function in the process of **metabolism.**

SUBACUTE. Midway between **acute** and **chronic** in the course of a disease.

SUSPENSION. A uniform mixture of insoluble fine particles in water or some other liquid. Liquid **antacids** are usually suspensions.

SUTURES. Stitches, clamps, or staples applied by a surgeon to hold the edges of a wound together until they heal.

SYMPATHETIC NERVOUS SYSTEM. (Derived from sympathin, the old name for adrenaline.) A network of nerves that trigger certain involuntary or automatic bodily functions, such as constricting blood vessels, making hair stand on end, raising "gooseflesh" on the skin, widening the pupils, contracting most **sphincters,** and speeding up the heartbeat. These stimuli add up to the "startle reaction" by which the body mobilizes for "fight or flight" in the face of sudden danger or surprise. (See also **central nervous system, parasympathetic nervous system.**)

SYMPTOM. What the patient complains of—from bad breath to palpitations to pain. A symptom is your body's signal to you that something is wrong (e.g., abdominal pain) and a clue to your doctor as to what its cause is likely to be. A sign is what your doctor finds on examination (e.g., tenderness of the abdomen). One sign or symptom is not a **syndrome,** but several signs and symptoms are.

SYMPTOMATIC RELIEF. The amelioration of **symptoms** of disease by such measures as the **administration** of medicine. For example, aspirin is commonly used for relief of pain, which is a symptom, rather than as treatment for the underlying cause of the pain.

SYNDROME. A set or constellation of **symptoms** or signs that together characterize or identify a specific disease or disorder.

SYNERGISTIC. The whole being greater than the sum of its parts. That is, when two or more effects applied at the same time multiply rather than add up their consequences. Thus, two **drugs** taken together may act synergistically—their effect is more than just the sum of each used separately.

SYSTEMIC. Referring to the body as a whole, rather than to **one** of its parts.

THERAPEUTIC EQUIVALENT. A **drug** that can be substituted for another without loss of efficacy.

THERAPY. Any form of medical treatment.

THROMBOSED. Refers to a vein or artery being plugged or clogged with clotted blood. When the thrombus (or clot) breaks loose and travels to another organ it is called an embolus and results in an embolism.

TIMED-RELEASE. A form of medication in which the active **drug** is purportedly absorbed into the bloodstream gradually over an extended period. Actually, the release rate may be highly variable from person to person and dose to dose.

TOLERANCE. The process by which the body adjusts to the effects of a **drug** and thus requires increased or more frequent dosages to achieve the desired effects. (See also **addicting, rebound effect.**)

TONE. A steady state of "stretch" or tension in healthy muscles enabling them to be always ready to respond rapidly to stimuli. Certain diseases diminish this normal tonicity, rendering muscles **atonic.**

TOPICAL. Applied directly on the skin (or accessible **mucous membrane**) to treat a **lesion** at its local site, rather than administered systemically (i.e., throughout the body, by way of the bloodstream or digestive tract).

TOURNIQUET. A cord, cloth, or something similar twisted around a wounded limb to stop blood loss. This old-time first-aid standby is now rarely recommended. Hand pressure or a pressure bandage is usually as effective, and far safer.

TOXIC. Poisonous: Effect ranging from harmful to lethal, depending on the dose taken and the resistance of the individual. (See also **detoxify.**)

TRANQUILIZER. A **drug** used to relieve anxiety and to calm. Major tranquilizers are used to treat **psychoses;** minor tranquilizers are used to relieve **symptoms** of anxiety and, sometimes, to relieve emotional stress associated with **organic disease.** Because it is less likely to produce drowsiness, a tranquilizer may be preferable to a **sedative,** particularly for daytime use.

TRIMESTER. The first, second, or third three-month period of the nine months of pregnancy.

TROCHE. A pill or lozenge that is dissolved in the mouth.

TUMOR. An abnormal growth on or in the body, which serves no useful purpose. A tumor may be malignant (cancerous) or benign (noncancerous).

URETHRA. A narrow channel (shorter in women than in men) through which the bladder voids urine. When the urethra is narrowed, as may happen with recurrent infection, it may have to be surgically stretched (dilated) to restore outflow.

UROLOGY. A branch of surgery dealing with the urinary tract—kidneys, ureters, bladder, **urethra**—plus (in males) the prostate gland and genitals.

USP. Refers to a **drug** compounded according to the *United States Pharmacopeia,* a semiofficial **pharmacological** directory of drug standards and specifications, issued every five years by a national committee of physicians, pharmacists, and academicians. (See also **NF.**)

VACCINE. A specially formulated mix of a weakened or killed **infection**-causing **bacterium** or **virus** introduced into the body so that the body through its immune mechanism will develop **antibodies** against the same bacterium or virus. These antibodies serve as protection against infection with the naturally occurring bacterium or virus.

VAPORIZER. A device for adding moisture or humidity to the air of a room. A cool-mist model does this by atomizing water into microdroplets. An electrolytic vaporizer boils water to steam up the atmosphere. A boiler-type vaporizer is also available.

VARICOSE VEINS. Abnormal veins that have become permanently stretched. There is an increased tendency for blood flow to slow down and for clots to form in these veins. Varicose veins usually occur in the legs and the anal region.

VASCULAR. Having to do with the blood's delivery system —arteries, veins, and **capillaries.**

VASOCONSTRICTOR. A chemical substance that narrows or shrinks the diameter of arteries and thereby reduces blood supply to an organ or tissue.

VASOMOTOR. Concerning or affecting the mechanism by which the walls of blood vessels expand and contract to regulate blood flow, blood pressure, and body temperature.

VECTOR. Anything that transmits **infection** from one **host** to another. Thus, a mosquito is the vector of malaria; a kiss (actually saliva) may be a vector of the common cold.

VIRUS. This smallest of all **microorganisms** causes a variety of viral **infections,** from fever blisters and German measles to poliomyelitis. Some viruses are suspected of triggering certain cancers. A virus causes havoc by invading a cell, disrupting its internal functioning, and distorting its reproduction mechanism.

WHITE BLOOD CELLS. Cells in the bloodstream that fight off **infection** by harmful **microorganisms.** One kind of white cell actually attacks **bacteria.** The other kind helps by making **antibodies.** Dead white cells and tissue, along with killed bacteria, collect as pus. (See also **serum factors.**)

WITHDRAWAL. See **addicting.**

Product index

General index